FROM CITY LIGHTS TO OUTBACK NIGHTS

A MIDWIFE'S EXTRAORDINARY JOURNEY THROUGH THE PANDEMIC

TERESA FREWEN

Copyright © 2024 TERESA FREWEN

The rights of Teresa Frewen to be identified as the author of the work has been asserted by her in accordance with the Copyright Act of Australia, 1968.

All rights reserved.

No part of this book may be reproduced or transmitted in any form or by any means, electronic or mechanical, including photocopying, recording or by any information storage and retrieval system, without prior permission in writing from the publisher.

For any enquiries or permissions, the publisher can be contacted at teresawalsh@hotmail.co.uk

First published in Australia by: Teresa Frewen

First Print: 2024

ISBN [Paperback]: 978-0-9-756515-5-1

CONTENTS

Acknowledgments   ix
Foreword   xiii
Author's Note   xvii

1. Benalla - Australia for a holiday in BC (Before Covid)   1
2. Fires, then the plague   4
3. Storm   9
4. Holiday in Australia   13
5. Small hospital bureaucracy   16
6. Stuck in Australia   27
7. Kangaroos at dawn   33
8. Norseman or Horseman   39
9. The Nullarbor   42
10. Australia's longest straightest road   44
11. Road train   50
12. Halfway across Australia   54
13. Priscilla Queen of the Desert   57
14. Quarantine In Alice Springs   67
15. Mparntwe, Alice Springs   73
16. Midwifery in Alice - An Ethical dilemma   75
17. Simpsons Gap, Mini Trips Out of Town   80
18. Ekala   87
19. Situational friendships   89
20. Kings Canyon camping   95
21. The Prisoner...things you see that you wish you hadn't.   103
22. Karlu Karlu - Getting away from it all   106
23. Tenant Creek   112
24. Weird and wonderful people and places   117
25. Tennant Creek Communities   125
26. WA Border Opening   139
27. Wealth   149
28. Canarvon   152

29. Metro midwife in Perth — 155
30. Did that just happen? — 161
31. Still stuck in Australia — 166
32. On the road again: Perth to Fitzroy Crossing — 175
33. Back to Work — 181
34. Fires, Plague, then Floods. — 184
35. Covid stone and Covid grey — 194
36. A Day in the life of a midwife - Fitzroy Style — 199
37. Good Friday Fitzroy Crossing — 204
38. Wangkatjungka clients — 210
39. ANZAC Day 2021 — 218
40. Calling it a day — 227
41. New Zealand's biggest lottery — 247
42. That feeling a midwife gets — 251
43. The journey continues — 258
44. Resignation again — 259
45. Reminders that I am a midwife — 261
46. Post Script — 276

Notes — 279

Jeff

I am forever grateful to you for turning up in your trusty Toyota at Fitzroy Crossing... and look where it got us!

I dedicate this book to my Highgate creative writing group, who were a constant connection during my time in Australia. We kept the writing muscle exercised and continue to do so every Wednesday.

With special thanks to Joyce (who was born before the Queen), and is my Highgate neighbour and writing companion. She continues to inspire me by publishing her books of poetry.

Extra special dedication to the late Valerie who was horrified at the thoughts of snakes, spiders and frogs and living in the desert, but encouraged me endlessly to keep writing about them.

ACKNOWLEDGMENTS

I would like to acknowledge the Traditional Custodians of the land on which I have worked and pay my respects to their Elders past and present. I extend that respect to Aboriginal and Torres Strait Islander peoples, especially the women who have shared their pregnancy journey with me.

In writing this book I would also like to acknowledge:

The Mercenaries who remind me that being motivated by money alone doesn't always end well.

The Misfits who have been a constant source of stories.

The Missionaries who remind me that there are still good people in the world and of course...

The Midwives who strive to be with women in the most challenging environments.

All these are people I have met on my journey as I went from working in the bustling city lights of London to the remote red dust plains of Australia.

Disclaimer

The following book recounts the experiences of a midwife travelling through Australia during the Covid-19 pandemic and her encounters with Australian Aboriginal places, people, and their way of life. The author has made every effort to provide accurate and respectful representations of Aboriginal culture and traditions, but it is important to acknowledge that Indigenous perspectives may differ from the author's own.

It is also important to note that Aboriginal people and communities have suffered from historical and ongoing injustices, including colonisation, forced removal from their lands, and cultural appropriation. The author acknowledges and condemns these injustices and recognises the importance of Indigenous voices in sharing their own stories and experiences.

This book is intended to promote cultural understanding and appreciation, but readers should approach the content with an open mind and recognise the complexities and nuances of Aboriginal culture and history. The author encourages readers to engage with Aboriginal people and communities in a respectful and supportive manner and to seek out additional resources for further education and understanding.

This book contains stories and characters that are written from the author's perspective. While some of the events and people portrayed in this book may be based on real-life experiences and individuals, all names and identifying characteristics have been changed to protect their privacy and anonymity.

The author acknowledges that some readers may find the stories and characters depicted in this book to be familiar or relatable to their own experiences. However, it is important to note that the stories and characters in this book are fictionalised and do not necessarily represent real-life people or events.

The author has taken great care to ensure that the characters and events portrayed in this book are not offensive or disrespectful to any particular individual or group. However, the author recognises that some readers may have different perspectives and experiences that may not align with those portrayed in this book.

Readers should approach the content of this book with an open mind and understand that the stories and characters presented are written from the author's perspective. The author does not intend to make any definitive statements or provide any solutions or answers to the issues and experiences portrayed in this book.

The author encourages readers to engage in critical thinking and reflection when reading this book and to seek out additional resources and perspectives for a more comprehensive understanding of the topics and themes discussed.

FOREWORD

I first met Teresa in 2017 in Mesen, Belgium when we were both there as part of the services to commemorate the centenary of the Battle of Messines. Teresa was there as part of the Ngāti Rānana London Māori Club which was playing a significant role in the WWI centennial services that had commenced in 2014. After a day of poignant services, a large group of Kiwis ended up socialising in Ypres. Like me, Teresa had been involved in the Parents Centre and in childbirth education so we had much in common to talk about. I was fascinated by Teresa's path as a New Zealander into Irish midwifery and her life and work in London, including her strong involvement in Ngāti Rānana. We became friends and have remained in touch.

Through social media, I followed Teresa's enforced and extended stay because of Covid in Australia, working as a contract nurse and midwife in Australia's vast outback. She wrote about places that I could never know and am unlikely to ever visit, just places on a map to me. I also knew of her extreme frustration with the MIQ system that had been introduced by the New Zealand government to restrict the numbers of those returning to New Zealand. To those Kiwis who were unable to return to their homeland to reconnect with families, the MIQ lottery was both unfeeling and unfair.

Teresa's story brings her Australian and Covid experiences to life. She could be a travel writer, with her descriptions of Australian outback making it easy to visualise its beauty, isolation, ruggedness and uniqueness. She also makes the potential dangers of driving in the vastness and loneliness of the outback seem very real and requiring both a sense of adventure and more than a little courage and perhaps foolhardiness. Fortunately, caring friends and relations prepared her well for her driving adventures.

Teresa's descriptions of the outback and its settlements are compelling – at times attractive, companionable and welcoming and at others repellant, unfeeling and unfriendly. I could sense how the vastness and isolation of the outback shapes people for better and for worse. The permanent residents have become inured to the comings and goings of the contracted workers and many of the measures they have adopted to deal with these make newcomers feel unwelcome and unappreciated. As a result, they bond much more readily with fellow transients although at times, this can be very testing, given the different personalities.

Teresa's empathy for and understanding of the aboriginal women, for whom she provides care, is very evident. It is difficult to read her accounts of the aboriginal settlements and the experiences of the aboriginal women in their pregnancy and birthing journeys without feeling frustrated and angry at a system that provides essential care but in such a flawed, disjointed, mechanistic way. It seems that the women are doomed to remain in a cycle of poverty and ill health and that this is the future for their children. It is easy to say everyone has choices in life but as Teresa relates, for these women these are only Hobson's choices. They have so little control over their lives or their futures and must live and die within health, education and social systems that are alien to their own culture.

It is interesting to read how Covid impacted Teresa's day to day life and her plans. All of us had to endure the restrictions that were imposed to deal with Covid but from the comfort and familiarity of our own homes and communities. To be in a large country for a much longer time than planned and to be constrained not only by international and national rules but those of different states whose borders you need to cross as Teresa did, was obviously an often frustrating experience, one associated with powerlessness and helplessness. In the way she describes it, it opens the reader to a quite different experience of the pandemic.

During my more than forty years' involvement in maternity services as a consumer, advocate and midwifery regulator, the midwives I have come to admire exhibit many qualities – amongst them tenacity, courage, humour, empathy, compassion and curiosity – as they are "with women" during their pregnancies, labour and birth and postnatal periods. I have certainly come to understand that midwifery is both a science and an art and the best midwives are those ones who bring those qualities to their work.

It is very evident as I read Teresa's account of her work and experiences in Australia that she possesses these qualities. She understands what it is to be "with women" in their pregnancy and birthing experience and that they, no matter what their socio-economic or cultural backgrounds are, deserve the best care a midwife can offer. I now look at the map which shows the vastness and apparent emptiness of interior Australia through a different lens.

A great read. I'm so pleased Teresa has taken the time and opportunity to share her *City Lights to Outback Nights* experience.

Sharron Cole
    Former President and Chair, Parents Centres New Zealand
    Former CEO, Midwifery Council of New Zealand

AUTHOR'S NOTE

Here's an idea if you are in a bit of a rut - you resign from your well-paid midwifery job in a very posh hospital in the middle of the UK capital (you know the one where the rich and famous go, and some Royal family members too), then fly halfway around the world to arrive in Australia and drive thousands of miles across that island continent caring for people living in the great Australian bush hundreds of miles from any reasonably populated town. Instead of looking after the Royals and film stars, you live and love your life with the locals and the first nations people.

There will be flies and frogs, snakes and dead kangaroos. You can't just go to this kind of place for a few months. You need to stay a couple of years at least. You will have to deal with droughts and floods, plagues and fires. You won't be alone, there will be all sorts of weird and wonderful people there. You might even fall in love. Who knows? What have you got to lose?

Nobody actually said this to me of course; and if they had, I would have baulked at the idea. But as life has a way of throwing us surprises, this is what I did.

Not quite by choice; but by accident.

London was my home: my adopted home, a city where I was happy. As a midwife, I had stepped out of the functional chaos of the NHS (National Health Service) and into the private sector, for a breather. There I stayed, caring for international women, expats from India, America, Australia and the Arab states; people with money or a job with good private health cover. Close to Europe, my boast was that I could catch the 214 TFL Transport for London bus, hoping to have Ahmed Serhani the friendliest bus driver, take me from the corner at Highgate to St Pancras International Train station, where I would board the Eurostar with a carry-a-board bag I didn't have to weigh, then pop up in Belgium, France or the Netherlands all within three and a half hrs.

As a new divorcee, I embraced this freedom, frequently. I was a Kiwi in London living my dream.

I had a delightful flat in Highgate village with one bedroom, bathroom and kitchen refashioned in the wardrobe; truly Londonesque with a separate 80's furnished lounge with a sofa big enough for friends or children to bunk on - but not comfortable enough for them to stay too long.

An hour north on the M1 was my narrowboat, rescued and in the throes of a refurbishment but comfortable enough to relax on the calming waters of the Nene. It was a perfect writing retreat.

My life was full, yet as 2018 was nearing the end, I was tired; not of London, but tired.

It had been a challenging year on both personal and professional levels.

I welcomed the New Year of 2019 with a gaggle of Italians who had embarked on a Speak programme, an English Language immersion. An equal mix of English speakers to Italian learners, I spent eight glorious days at Abbazia de Spineto. This unique Abbey provides 800 hectares of incredible landscape in the Val d'Orcia,

Tuscany, blending tradition with an astonishing collection of design masterpieces.

The Anglos in the group had to speak English and my thick New Zealand accent was a challenge for many. The Italians had to speak English as well. That is what they had signed up for. It was a most blessed and healing environment for me set amidst the picturesque Tuscan hills eating seasonal Italian cuisine and drinking the local Vino Nobile wines.

Infused with motivation and creativity, feeling the ghosts of the monks in the rooms and corridors of the former holy place, I came to know what I needed to do during the year ahead. I was mentally prepared for my life change. I planned to step away from London for six months, go to Australia for some sunshine, and then return fresh ready to direct my energy full time into my fledgling business, Newborninthecity ™.

On April 1, 2019, I sat the IBCLC exam in the exam centre in Holburn, UK. Part of my plan was to become an International Board Certified Lactation Consultant, a coveted certificate for which I had studied ridiculously hard before I left.

I stepped out of that exam looking up to the tower blocks of central London knowing I was destined for change.

That day, I booked my return flight from London to Melbourne and told my four adult children and selected friends about my plans to go to Australia.

Some thought I was brave, many thought I would not come back. My adult kids rallied in support. I would miss Ellen's visit to London, but I would see her in Wellington in March. Hannah would look after my car and use it for driving practice; Vinny would sublet my flat "only for six months though Mum, you can't stay any longer" and Ted and Liva cleared the sofa in Melbourne, which was like my London one - not too comfortable.

I would take my time to leave and plan for an endless summer. It is often the way that when you decide to leave a place, you see all that is good. It was this way for me even though I knew I was only going for six months. I had a fabulous few months tripping to Ireland, hosting with the New Zealand Pilgrimage Trust a hikoi to the Western Front in Belgium as a commemoration to Ngati Ranana's 60th anniversary. Taking in all that is good about London, meeting with friends and going to a Hanson concert. I met Ray Davies from the Kinks and sang along with Gordon Lightfoot in the Round House – from the seats of course.

I took every opportunity to see parts of the UK and finally went to the Isle of Wight.

A reunion with my *Speak Italian* friends was my final hurrah. On a Saturday morning outside a Café, in a cobbled street in the Town of Matera region of Basilicata, surrounded by Italians who didn't really know much about rugby, a group of South African Mining executives on a junket, I watched the All Blacks defeated by England in the RWC2019.

My Italian friends baked a cake with 'Happy Travels Teresa' piped into the icing.

The fact that I would be in Melbourne the following week, softened the reality that the All Blacks had lost.

I had already secured a midwifery contract in the state of Victoria before leaving the UK. Having lived in Australia before made this an easier task than for many who want to head down under to work. Thankfully, I had faithfully paid The Australian Health Practitioner Regulation Agency (AHPRA) each year, often wondering if I would ever need it again.

But here I was.

1 BENALLA - AUSTRALIA FOR A HOLIDAY IN BC (BEFORE COVID)

I had dealt with my jet lag and my tenure on the sofa was up. My son Ted, drove me up the highway to my new home in what seemed like a parent-child reversed role. My shared accommodation consisted of a two-bedroom self-contained flat with an outside area. The child-size single bed was an eye-rolling surprise; but for whatever reason, that was the way it was in Benalla. The apartment was cleaned every week. My flatmate worked in Medical Records but was on a long holiday in Japan; so, I was not to expect her until early in the new year. Apart from the single bed, it was a fantastic accommodation, with efficient aircon and only a five-minute cycle to work.

Benalla Hospital is 200 km northeast of Melbourne. It is considered a 'rural placement' and can facilitate low-risk birthing. There are midwives and GPOs who are General Physicians with further training in Obstetrics. I had taken up a contract for four months and would travel back to Melbourne on the slow and unreliable train on my days off, visiting my son, Ted and his wife, Liva. The hospital was small, the people were friendly. It is the cleanest hospital I have ever worked in and I am still in contact with a couple of the women who run the cleaning dept. The birth rate was slowing down year by year, but enough to keep the service for the local women in that area.

This hospital had a positive vibe, but it was still a challenge to attract midwifery staff.

On a two-day break, close to Christmas, I visited Melbourne. My son and his wife were both working, so we met for a Christmas feast with matching wines as only these two hospitable humans could perfect.

I visited my deliciously eccentric Aunty Bee in Geelong. We met one of my younger cousins for the first time as adults. I introduced him to Aperol Spritz and we ate pavlova baked with the Edmonds cookbook recipe (a New Zealand icon). Back in Melbourne, I met up with my nephew from Taranaki for a taste of local beers.

It was a blessed couple of days.

I had been living in Benalla for all of two months and found being in the city was refreshing and invigorating, yet I was slightly disconnected as I had gotten so used to the darkness of the Northern hemisphere and Christmas lights which had become a beacon of hope during the dreary winter nights.

Here, in the balmy Australian heat, clear blue skies and high temperatures, the decorations and lights seemed impotent.

I was very happy to work Christmas, so the local midwives could spend time with their families. Benalla welcomed a Christmas Eve baby, and they went home on Christmas day. Santa was very clever in that family.

In the hospital, as part of the festive season, a broom cupboard had been transformed into Santa's grotto, adorned with tinsel and lights and a crazy dancing Santa. Staff brought their families up to the grotto. It was good fun.

At lunchtime, on the 25th wearing my Santa hat and Christmas earrings, I joined the ward staff for dinner. They had a formally set table with crackers, doilies and table decorations. The cooks served us a roast dinner and plum pudding.

I called my colleague to delay her start time and she arrived mid-afternoon. I had watched an episode or two of 'Father Ted' on the computer. There were no phone calls, no labouring mums. The ED was without emergencies and the handful of patients in the ward were resting. Outside the sky was blue, the Jacaranda tree had shed her flowers to transform the ground beneath into a carpet of purple petals.

All was calm.

A million miles from the snow clad village of Oberndorf and its *Silent Night* carol, all was calm, a different kind of calm

I was not prepared for the fires, nor the plague.

2 FIRES, THEN THE PLAGUE

I had always known that Australia had fires. I remember as a child in Southland, New Zealand, seeing the smoky hue in the sky from bushfires. This was wondrous to a child for whom Australia was a country, a very long way away. It fascinated me; I knew it was something ominous.

When I started in Benalla, I always noticed the fire blanket and other safety equipment in the boot of the pool car we used for work, but it was not until New Year's Eve, that I realised why it was a necessary kit.

It was the fire season. Australia defines itself in seasons: wet season, dry season, fire season. The news went from mentioning the latest outbreaks, to headlining the special reports as the disaster worsened. The familiar face of Shane Fitzsimmons who was the Fire commissioner for New South Wales became a household name and the mesmerising voice of the disaster that came over the radio and television several times a day, seemed to be inching closer and closer as the fire began reaching uncharted territory.

There were pictures of dystopian ruins where country settlements had burned to the ground. The skeletal-like chassis of cars whose occupants had miraculously escaped, and homes completely untouched by neither heat nor flame appeared side by side on our screens with the charred stems of trees and shrubs. From the comfort of my lounge, it both fascinated and terrified me how indiscriminate the fire was; how calm and determined many of the homeowners remained, some refusing to leave, putting the firefighters at risk, all to stay home right till the last minute. The fire department had long been urging them to flee with their family and pets. But who knows what their reasons were to make them stay put and put lives in danger?

Television footage of the little koalas with their paws and bums burned raced all over the internet. It was heartbreaking.

For days, the smell and taste of smoke were a constant reminder of the devastation happening in Victoria and New South Wales. They have gone down in history as the Black Summer Bushfires of 2019-2020.

We all had a fire warning app which updated us of risky areas and would ping if pre-populated areas of interest came under threat.

Evidence carried across the sky left a dirty cloudy haze. In the evenings, the setting sun looked like an eerie unnatural orange ball hanging low in the sky. Through the trees, it reminded me of the midwinter dull light the northern hemisphere experiences.

The heaviness was smoke. It tasted and smelled like a bonfire.

I learned about fire preparedness, evacuation plans, stay and protect, and pack and wait.

I was always in a state of slight alertness, keeping an eye not only on my own area but also on the locations of my family members in the city. It amazed me how calm everyone seemed to be. I followed the news closely, shocked by the images of burning buildings and the fierce, orange-red flames. The fires were truly powerful.

The staff at the hospital were affected too. In this rural town, it was a common occurrence for employees to be absent, as everyone knew who lived near the fire hot spots. The local staff stepped up and covered shifts for their absent colleagues.

Some of our pregnant mothers adjusted their prenatal appointments, which was understandable, but overall, the unit continued to operate as usual.

Shift patterns vary from hospital to hospital across Australia, and here in Benalla, they had a built-in 'double staff time' of two hours overlapping with morning and afternoon shifts. This was to facilitate handover, lunch breaks, home visits, education, and fire updates. This is invaluable and what I consider should be protected time, especially when it is one midwife per shift. Not all hospitals facilitate this, and often agency staff are asked not to start until the last minute. Benalla used the double time well.

A domiciliary (Dom) midwife home visit is provided for, under maternity care in Australia. The exact number of visits changes from state to state and will depend on staff availability and then client needs. It has always been an aspect of midwifery care that I love.

My business in London focused on providing postnatal support to women in their homes, as this environment allows for a more collaborative partnership. I was in Benalla without a car, so I often volunteered to do home visits to keep myself busy and to pick up any heavy or frozen grocery items. This was an unofficial arrangement, but I always made sure to do it on my own time.

On one home visit, I was scheduled to meet a new mother and her baby who had recently returned from giving birth in Melbourne. I set the navigation system and headed to their home, which was about an hour east of Benalla. I was able to enjoy the scenic drive, and the cloudy smoky haze that day was less threatening than it had been on previous days.

When I arrived at the patient's house, I found that it was located 25 km off the main road, up a winding dirt track on their well-signed property. As I pulled in, I noticed that their vehicle was packed as if the family were about to go on a month-long holiday. In reality, they were preparing to evacuate because of a nearby fire. The father, a farmer, was still out fighting the fire, but they had been given the all-clear to stay put. I was completely unaware of the danger and only realised in hindsight that I was not prepared to face a fire.

Apparently, I should never have driven out to the patient's home. I was unaware of these regulations, and my manager scolded me, in a casual but dismissive manner

It's possible that there may come a day when midwives are required to have a competency in fire appreciation.

The 2019-20 bushfires in Victoria and New South Wales destroyed more than 300 homes and almost 7000 head of stock. There were over 1.5 million hectares of public and private land much of which were forests and parks, plantations and native forests, critical animal habitats and water catchment areas that were touched by the fires.

On a summer Thursday, after the fire threat had diminished, I had two home visits scheduled. The first visit was at the back of a takeaway restaurant. As I was speaking with the new mother about breast engorgement and diaper contents, a man entered the room and offered me a cold bottle of water and a serving of freshly cooked charcoal chicken and chips as a gesture of gratitude for visiting the shop owners and their new baby.

I hadn't realised they owned the business. It's not what you know but who you know in Benalla - and now I know the best take away - of course, the baby and mum were doing fine! And I did finish my check.

What a treat! The hot chips and aircon had lulled me into a false sense of complacency as I drove about an hour to my second and last visit of the afternoon. It was a rural district called Tatong, with rolling straw-coloured lands and clumps of trees punctuating colour into the dry farms. Skinny looking cows could be seen grazing on the deep roots that apparently have good nutrition.

Tatong happens to have been the birthplace of Michael Joseph Savage, a famous Prime Minister of New Zealand, who led the first Labour government from 1935 until his death in 1940. I had learned about him in school and recalled that he was known to be the architect of the welfare state. There is a memorial to him in Tatong. I relish finding interesting pieces of history in the most surprising places even when providing a midwifery service in rural Australia.

I grew up in a very remote part of the southern hemisphere. Not the Antarctic, but close enough to have Aurora Australis as a childhood norm. It is a cold province. It would be common enough for the weather to be 4-6 degrees even in summer; so, when I saw that the outside temperature was 46 deg centigrade in Australia that day, it seemed a peculiar juxtaposition of the numbers.

Maybe the thermometer was broken? 46degC? Surely not? Unbelievable. But officially correct.

Eventually, I found the right farmhouse, and as I opened the door it was as though I was entering an oven.

The heat was indescribable and there were a zillion flies. I made a dash towards the fly-free zone of the house.

For the first time in my midwifery career, after fighting my way through a veil of flies, I went straight in through the backdoor without waiting for the household to answer my knock. The family whom I knew from their birthing and stay in Benalla were gracious and understanding. Along with a nicely brewed tea, our postnatal check was completed.

All was well in the house with the mum and new-born. Grandmother knew of Highgate, in London well and as the whole family were planning a wedding trip to Norfolk in April we had an idea to meet up in London - dependent of course on the Corona Virus situation. There were murmurings of travel disruption.

I thought it would be lovely to see one of my Ozzie babies in London.

I felt a little homesick.

Safely home and reflecting back from the comfort of my aircon unit faithfully running 24/7 and paid for by Benalla Health, I realised that my sabbatical in Australia was going to be full of surprises - the kind I had not ever anticipated.

3 STORM

During a morning shift, I had the privilege of caring for three mothers and their newborns. After the shift ended, I invited a colleague over for a meal and since I had just won a raffle for fresh fruit and vegetables at the golf club, I decided to cook a meal for us. I needed to purchase some meat, so I drove (using a car borrowed from work) to the local Aldi store.

While I was at the store, I received a call from my son in Melbourne, who was 200 km away. He asked about the weather, and I laughed and told him it was lovely, with a cooler temperature than the previous day, now only 39 degrees Celsius. On the other end of the line, I could hear the rain pouring down in Melbourne and as we said goodbye, I reminded him to stay safe.

Pulling into the mostly empty car park, I looked south in the direction of Victoria's capital, Melbourne, and I could see a cloudy, stormy, fiery sky that I had never seen before. Slightly pink from the red pindan sand, slightly grey from forest smoke, with an overlay of murky.

My tourist's eye thought it could have been a great photo, but then the first slash of lightning crackled across the sky just as I was about to click. It gave me a fright.

A couple entering the store made some comments about getting home quick. I wasn't overly worried, thinking it was the storm in Melbourne – miles away. And I still had the work vehicle.

Then, at the fresh meat counter, a noise deafened us. BOOM ! Then dark!

The power had gone out.

I had a cut of lamb in my hand which I needed for dinner. A check-out chick called rather urgently to the handful of customers "You all have to leave now".

"Can I just take this, and I'll pay tomorrow?" I asked.

"No, you have to go". She grabbed the lamb cutlets from my hand, leaving me no choice but to exit empty-handed.

I did wish I had just thrown it in my reusable bag and walked out. I had no meat for dinner.

Whether it was a storm, a tornado or a meteorological event, I was caught in the middle of something wild and terrifying. The drive only a few blocks to my flat was punctuated by flying shrubs, broken branches just missing the car, and dust so thick I couldn't actually see the road. Stopping and taking shelter was not an option.

Back in the safety of my home, I wasn't sure if my heart rate was elevated due to excitement or fear. I think it was a bit of both.

As quickly as it had arrived, the storm passed.

Eventually, my colleague made her way to my flat using a taxi to avoid the fallen tree across her road. She had a rescue supply of candles and torches. No electricity meant that dinner would need to be anything raw. I had a Prosecco and it was already chilled.

I always have Prosecco.

My colleagues knew I was very happy to do the domiciliary visits and on one occasion I may have gotten a little bit lost and found myself at Glenrowan, where the notorious Ned Kelly's standoff occurred.

Ned Kelly was a legendary bushranger whose gang of bandits held a fierce reputation for robbery and murder. His claim to fame was the ambushing and murder of three police officers who had attempted to arrest his brother, Dan. Ned was hunted down, convicted and executed in Melbourne on 11th November 1880.

A very large art form of him directs the tourists to the actual spot where weathered wooden statues of his gang and the police are all in position.

I saw a sign for Bailey's winery. I had been recommended to go there by the family I had just visited. Ned Kelly would have to wait.

I did get to the vineyard in time to taste and purchase a few bottles of locally grown 'grape juice' before safely delivering the work car back to the yard.

I thought to myself, "Today is altogether another day. It's raining."

Some parts of the country were flooding, as was - by coincidence - my hometown in NZ. But here in Australia, the mighty rain was falling, and the news was showing mankini-clad[1] farmers dancing in the streams, and dogs taking shelter from the unusual stuff falling from the sky as many had not ever felt rain in these regions. The fire commissioner was smiling in his daily interview on TV and the *fireys* (volunteer firefighters) were posting updates of themselves line dancing in the puddles.

Here in Benalla, I went to the art gallery for the first time. I had been saving this cultural experience for a rainy day. I was surrounded by middle-aged women who thought Botox was an improvement to their looks. Their dyed blond and weathered skin was as much a uniform as the local high school tunic. A far cry from the demographic of women I had met at the Midwifery unit. These women appeared to be wives of wealthy farmers or successful horse owners.

Looking at the vibrant colours of their clothes and the liberal use of dangly earrings and necklace art, I felt I could almost fit in. But I'm not blonde.

For the first time, I contemplated staying in the area, but quickly dismissed the notion. I was enjoying the pace of life and also found a delightful cinema in Swanpool, where at half time in the movie you were served tea and cakes.

Hospitality was plentiful in Benalla. One Sunday, after attending a coffee meet-up for new Benalla folk, I joined the local Anglican church for a floral and choral recital. I met Carol there. She was in her seventies and had composed a piece for the organ many years ago. That day was the first time she had played it in public. She was also an artist and invited me to the local painting group. There, I was a bit of a novelty but soon I learned all the women's gossip around Benalla and also heard how their babies had been born. Carol had had her five children at home.

I never tire of hearing the eloquence of birth memories. It is a reminder to me that how I care for and treat a woman when she is birthing, is never forgotten. They will forget my name, but not how I treated them.

Carol and I met for coffee most weeks. Then one day she didn't turn up. She had died very suddenly. Her funeral had happened, and it was one of the saddest pieces of news I had received in a long while. I am so glad she performed in the church that afternoon.

4 HOLIDAY IN AUSTRALIA

February 2020.

If I was to fly for four hours in Europe, I would have been flying internationally, across many countries and using my passport. My ticket leaving Melbourne airport was just to Perth. I had been curious to know if I could really board this flight using my driver's licence as ID, fly for almost four hours and disembark avoiding customs. *'Too easy,'* the catch cry of Victoria passed through my thoughts as I smiled and realised it was.

Australia is vast and even though I do know it in theory, it is a tangible reality when flying from coast to coast. I am a collector of Aboriginal art and looking out of the Qantas aircraft's window over the land below, I could see the curves floating through the sands carving designs that lift the eye and which are the dots of my art. It is said that the Aboriginal Dreamtime gives the perspective from above and this is how the art is imagined. I can see it. The water holes were now white with salt. The rivers' paths stretch beyond what the eye can see. The fertile clumps of green punctuate the barren lands. It is magic and the art is dynamic.

I lived and worked in Western Australia thirteen years ago. It was here I first encountered a cultural bias, as many Australians disliked Kiwis (New Zealanders) coming in and taking their jobs. In that very brief encounter, I had a penny-drop moment and it has formed my understanding of racist commentary ever since.

Unlike Benalla, there are Aboriginal people living in Western Australia. It was quietly reassuring that although they are a minority group clawing to get a voice, they are visible. In Benalla, the locals told me *they were all shot out* in such a matter-of-fact way that I couldn't respond.

Over in the West, it is very different and yet very Australian. Kangaroo are plentiful, quokkas, emu, snakes, pelican, liquorice ice-cream and Margaret River wine. The Swan river seduces the 'boaties' and the irrigation schemes keep the parks green. It is a place of pleasure. Except there is a poison that is starting to sour the taste buds of many. The plight of the indigenous population and the attempt to incorporate cultural traditions is leading to a rising prejudice.

As part of a commitment to redress wrongs, the Australian Federal Government issued an apology. On 13th February 2008, the then prime minister, Kevin Rudd formally apologised to Aboriginal and Torres strait islander peoples, especially to the Stolen Generations whose lives had been wronged by past government policies. Since then, a protocol where Aboriginal or Torres Strait Islander Traditional Owners welcome others to the land of their ancestors has been adopted. It is called Welcome to Country.[1]

The Welcome to Country ceremony is carried out at significant events and formal functions involving people from other parts of the country or from overseas. This practice shows respect for the Traditional Owners and Elders of a particular area or region.

The WARSL, Western Australia Return Serviceman's League, in their wisdom changed their rules and banned the welcome-to-country ceremony, in any language other than English or Maori during the NZ anthem, for the ANZAC ceremony this coming April. I was outraged when I read it, immediately posting it to my FB profile, wanting to spread incredible news to the world, even though I know my world is very small.

The sadness and outrage I felt were a surprise to my family who are well-settled in WA. The silence and lack of commentary showed me how ingrained the ignorance of first nations people's plight is. Australia is like that. I didn't see an ostrich, but feel that many locals do choose to bury their heads and there is plenty of sand to do so.

The RSL eventually retracted their plans. The rhetoric was clearly only to save face and nothing else. *'We only ask for two days'* (*that we don't have to do this shit*) is what they meant.

I vowed to be flying an aboriginal flag at ANZAC ceremony in Ypres on the Western Front this April, and I will speak Te reo maori (maori language) to show respect to all New Zealanders and support for the traditional landowners here in a country I am so grateful to be able to visit and work.

My time with my Whānau (family) was a tiny jewel, as I was going back to London, I said my good byes wondering when or if I would see them again.

5 SMALL HOSPITAL BUREAUCRACY

I thought about the day of the storm often. Of course, the highlight was the charcoal chicken, but as I drove through the dry and vast countryside, what struck me was the contrasting situations I found myself in during my stay in Australia. A few weeks from that visit, on a day that was not quite as extreme in temperature, I was on my way to another family, on another farm, in another district. This mum had been discharged from the special care baby unit (SCBU) in another hospital. She was a first-time mother of twins who still weighed less than two kilos.

The State of Victoria was in the shadows of the fire season. In the work vehicle, we kept a fire blanket and instruction sheet advising what to do if caught in a fire. To this day, I acknowledge that I hadn't realised the significance or real possibility of getting caught by fire. I remained naive and a little too Kiwi with my, "she'll be right" mentality.

The drive was, once again, into the vast countryside with mid-summer, brown landscapes and bumpy gravel roads. I pulled into a farm track and drove up to the house. Parked in front was a Landcruiser packed to the brim with items that would ordinarily be for a family holiday.

The mum, her parents - who were on holiday from Scotland - and the twins were all in the lounge. The adults were drinking tea and the babies were asleep in a single bassinet.

I joined them for tea. As a domiciliary midwife, information is gleaned from the overall maternal well-being as part of our visit. Over a cup of tea, I learned that the family had packed up the vehicle as part of a "prepare to evacuate" order. The helicopters had just left the back of their farm, which in fairness could have been many kilometres away, but the fire had been heading towards their home. However, it had just been put out and their risk had been downgraded. They would remain on alert. I didn't meet the dad. He would not be home much and the grandparents were doing a sterling job supporting their daughter and her twin babies. I got the feeling they were in a constant state of alert. It was their first visit to Australia during the summer months, which is also the fire season, and Grandad said it was the most excitement he'd had in years. He hoped there wouldn't be too much more though.

The twins had been weighed the day before by another service provided by the hospital-in-home team. This was initiated at the hospital where the babies were born. They had forgotten to inform us, or maybe they had; but the shared care/shared responsibility model was new to me. I assessed and initiated women's health physio care for the mum, who seemed to have been omitted from any post-natal assessments. I enquired about the feeding and behaviours of the twins over the previous 24 hrs and made a clinical decision not to wake the babies for a weigh-in. The hospital-in-home team were doing a final visit the next day and would discharge them from their books. I scheduled another domiciliary visit for the following week.

When I arrived back at the hospital, there was a message for me to call the hospital-in-home team and advise them of the babies' weights. I called them back and told them I hadn't weighed the babies. I was met with a stony, annoyed response and an accusatory attitude. I was indignant and the call ended with frosty vibes from the midwife at the other hospital. This phone call was closely followed by a visit from the acting DON(Director of Nursing), who carried on with the frosty rhetoric and questioned why I had not weighed the twins.

My clinical judgement was not what was expected. I was supposed to have weighed the twins because the hospital-in-home team needed to discharge the twins. I suspected it was about funding or the big brother hospital lording it over simple community service - 'confirming' that we were not able to do our job. To this day, I don't know what all the fuss was about. I remained indignant, and because I was right in my clinical midwifery assessment, they could not reprimand nor discipline me; but I could be forever labelled 'bolshy'. And so, I was. My colleague who was working in the clinic was directed to return to the home in the country, close to a 90-minute return journey plus consultation time, to weigh the babies. No logical rationale was ever offered. We made sure she was paid overtime. The acting DON was livid.

When my manager returned from leave, I was summoned to the office to discuss "the issue." As I had suspected, it was about funding and expectations of our service not being communicated. The big brother hospital was taking a stab at the country hospital by accusing our midwifery team of incompetence.

That's how it sometimes is in rural Australia.

Remote domiciliary visits are different in different states and hospitals. In Carnarvon, WA there was always an Aboriginal Liaison Officer (ALO). She would reliably know the family and where they would be on any given day. She would weigh the baby and I would check the mum. It was a delight to have her, and I felt there was a cultural acknowledgement that is essential for indigenous women. I felt more comfortable in the homes of Aboriginal and Torres Strait Islander people when accompanied by an ALO. In Tennant Creek, we didn't have ALOs, so our visits were solo; but more of those stories to come later.

I was seldom invited into the homes there, so I would at times, weigh the baby on the scales near the car. Blood pressure (BP) checks would be done while mum was standing and they would talk discreetly about womanly things that happened during birth, like blood loss. I called this opportunistic care. More commonly, I would pick them up and bring them to the hospital. We had a baby car seat permanently fixed in the work car. After the postnatal check, they would usually walk into town or get dropped off somewhere else. It was part of the deal in many ways. Although it was never an official Uber service, it sometimes felt like it. When the babies were six weeks old, they would visit the child health nurse (CHN) for the needles. We had a great system going and between the CHN and midwife, we would manage to track the mum and baby down. Immunisations and postnatal discharge from our service would be given.

I was nearing the end of my contract in Benalla. In the beginning, everyone and everything was new and, with all the best intentions, I had tried not to get caught up in the politics of the place. I had, however, figured out that the midwifery educator, who had not practised midwifery for years, got her position because she was in a relationship with one of the managers. That manager was on "stress leave" because the educator had had an affair with another staff member. The manager was lovely, but she reminded me of one of my teachers back in my Catholic school days. It turned out that she had actually been a Sister. I had also figured out who amongst the nursing staff was there because they had partners with steady work in the area, who were there because they didn't fit into the big city hospitals, and who, like me, were there just for the short-term contract. They worked hard, then left. I got the gist of which doctors did what and which doctors were easier to work with.

I had been introduced to a few nursing students but I was not impressed by what I saw.

On one late shift, I was working in the acute ward. An elderly gentleman was being transferred back to his nursing home where his wife, also living there, was waiting. This gentleman's life was nearing its end, so we were providing social palliative care.

I went to help two student nurses, who had been directed to assist the ambulance driver and get the patient transferred to the trolley. As it happened, the gentleman had incontinence that needed attention. Both students, in their final year, did not know how best to start cleaning this man in order to make his transfer possible. I got started, then thought "bloody hell these students have no idea," so I took off my gloves and apron and stepped back. I said, "I'm a midwife, and you are both student nurses. You take the lead and let me know if you need me to help."

To this day, I don't know if it was the incontinence or the fact that I made them use their initiative, but it took them some time to figure out what to do. As I ended that shift, I realised I was ready to get on with my plan in life. I was also looking forward to my holiday in New Zealand and getting back to London.

Little did I know what was ahead.

***

Accidentally in Australia

Coronavirus chaos started for me on the Saturday before the 17th of March 2020, St Paddy's day, which was to be my last shift at Benalla.

One of our mums came in labouring. It was her third baby and as is the custom in Benalla, I was in the unit on my own with the GP obstetrician on call. My colleague was coming in for the pm shift and if needed, I could call her in to start early.

As my client and her husband settled into their birthing room, I was aware of numerous vibrations coming from my mobile. Someone needed to get a hold of me and I was worried. I stepped out of the labour room, and saw notifications from my son in Melbourne and my daughter Ellen, in New Zealand. She had called three times. Ellen doesn't call.

Now I was really worried.

Ted's text was, "Seen the news?"

Ellen's text said, "I don't think you can come, mum! Call me."

She had sent a news clip from Jacinda Ardern (the then Prime Minister of NZ), hot off the press.

Coronavirus 19: Everyone entering New Zealand will be required to isolate. Cruise ships banned. It went on. This news had come directly from the cabinet committee meeting.

I was aware New Zealand had banned flights from China back in February, but now it was ramping up. NZ had just recorded its 6th case of coronavirus.

I had a three-week holiday booked and I had planned to spend some time with my eldest daughter Ellen, as well as take flights to Invercargill, Christchurch, Wellington, New Plymouth, Auckland, and the length and breadth of Aotearoa. I had lunch dates, tramping trips, drinks, sleepovers, reunions and real estate meetings planned. I would then bounce back to Australia to work in Melbourne for a month, with a flight back to 'old blighty' booked. I anticipated I would have some sunshine-infused enthusiasm left over to focus on revamping my new business venture, 'Newborninthecity ™' when back in London.

In a flash, each frame of my life plan, clear sequential and coordinated, was warped by time and the virus and seemed to be evaporating fast.

A few days earlier, the World Health Organisation had declared Coronavirus-19 a pandemic. I, like everyone, had been following the news and had an appreciation of the gravity of the situation. But I had assumed it would be isolated to other countries like SARS and Swine flu had been before. While working in London, we had to learn how to use PPE. New signage went up around the hospital and patients were screened for travel history. Midwives and Nurses had to practise wearing PPE and isolation rooms were prepared. We had become sceptical and blasé. This would be gone before it arrived.

My text reply to both of my kids was, "busy birthing the newest Ozzie baby, I'll call later." I turned my phone off and went back to the mum who was labouring.

The magic that is birthing, meant I was able to completely disengage from the outside world that had just taken a giant U-turn.

Baby S was born and placed onto her mother's chest, umbilical cord still attached and pulsing to pass on the last of the goodness from the placenta into her little body. As she took her first breath, you could see her dad's broad farming shoulders soften with relief. He cried the most wholesome tears as he stared at his beautiful, baby girl.

I also cried a discrete tear and wondered what world this newest baby was being born into. Baby S weighed in at 3630 grams. She was 52 cm long with a head circumference of 36 cm. She was born at 14:46 on the day New Zealand closed its international borders. The day I couldn't go home.

In midwifery circles, we dance around the terms we use when a baby is born.

Does the midwife birth the baby (doesn't the mother)? Does she deliver it? (No; a pizza is delivered). Does she catch the baby? What if she drops it?

Whatever the fad or correct term on the endless paperwork is, my name is recorded as the accoucheur for the purpose of registering the birth.

It is very unlikely that this lovely mum will say, "Oh, Teresa was my accoucheur." I imagine she will just simply say, "Teresa delivered my baby." Like I say, "Sister Spiers delivered me all those years ago in Bluff."

I waded through the paperwork. I declined to hand it over to my colleague and completed all the legal documentation and clinical records of the labour and birth myself; perhaps with more detail than was required.

Deep down, I was avoiding facing the changing landscape of my life.

I didn't turn on my phone until I was home, showered and dried, and poured myself a large brandy.

Shaken not stirred, I got straight onto the Air New Zealand site and their customer hotline first thing Monday morning. To their credit, I was refunded in full for all the international and national flights. This was after a rather protracted, but calm insistence that as a Londoner, I couldn't use credit and although I would happily transfer the credits to my daughter, legally this was not possible. When the staff member finally succumbed to the pressure (she did actually understand but everything was such a mess in the Air New Zealand offices) she said, "I'm just going to do it. I'm not supposed to, but I get it. Just don't tell anyone. The money will be in your bank within 48 hours."

And so, it was. I never did tell anyone how amazing Air New Zealand was in this matter. For many others that followed, the process was not so straightforward. I stayed schtum.

I became more Irish than the Irish on my last day at Benalla and we drank a Guinness while bestowing the luck of the Irish to my midwifery colleagues and the new friends I had made in this lovely provincial town in Victoria.

Plan B had not been imagined and pandemic variance was a challenge. My son and his wife lived in a one-room apartment in Melbourne, so I needed to find somewhere else to stay. My aunty Be, generous in her open house offer, was 'health vulnerable' so I couldn't take up either of these offers.

London flights were cancelled as well. The world was closing.

Both my siblings again welcomed their little sister into the WA fold. I booked a flight to Perth, the second in as many months.

Instead of looking down over the Southern Alps, Aoraki, or Aspiring, what I saw from the aeroplane was an expanse of brown with the occasional irrigated green patch and the never-ending countryside of Australia.

The world's core was heating up and there was an eggshell climate of uncertainty.

The news told me that Italy was desperate and the velvet curtains of coronavirus were being drawn ever so slowly in London.

The shutters of protection slammed shut on Aotearoa, New Zealand.

Hour by hour, the vapour trails vanished, the rules changed; the toilet paper disappeared.

It would be the last time, for some time, that I could hug my son, as I took the intrepid steps to board the flight to Perth. The Melbourne departure terminal had a smattering of mask-wearing travellers weaving back and forth, unimpeded along the queue gates.

Cancelled. Cancelled. Cancelled. The once spectacular wish list destinations were rapidly draining hope from travellers' hearts.

The news channels stated that a staggering two-thirds of the Qantas staff had already been stood down from duty. I bought boxes of lovely Belgian chocolates.

The plane was almost empty. The gratitude I felt is unquantifiable and the chocolates seemed pathetic, but I gave them to the onboard staff, said I was sorry, and remained grateful.

The simple gesture paid off. I wasn't quite upgraded, but they plied me with first-class wine in proper glasses. It was great!

My big brother was surprised at just how chatty his sister could be, when plied with alcohol, but happy to see me. In the beginning of the Coronavirus -19 outbreak, the Commonwealth and state government officials were making up rules on the hop. There were lockdowns, restrictions, and closures. International statistics should have alerted everyone to sit up and take notice. History will write its own account, as Australia and New Zealand seemed to be impervious to the mass devastation, by simply hanging up the closed sign.

WA didn't seem to have noticed that there was a pandemic.

It was here I was intrigued that I could not smell the frangipanis on my walk around the river and estuary of Pelican Point which is where my brother lived. It was some months later that anosmia was listed as a symptom of covid.

I had friends in London who were very unwell but testing for coronavirus wasn't a thing. Politically, the tests were only available to the public if they presented to a hospital with viral symptoms. My niece, a young dietitian, was deployed within the largest London trust Guy's and St Thomas' and although she was really crook[1], was not able to screen and therefore was never counted in the statistics. She suffered long Covid symptoms for many months and eventually left London. Something was happening out in the world. It was called a pandemic but few, including myself, thought it would come to much in the developed world.

After all, Australia was a long way from the epicentre.

WA sleep walked through the lockdown by closing restaurants and hairdressers but keeping hardware, garden, and some other major brand shops open. To me, it seemed as if it was life as usual in sleepy Bunbury where I stayed for the duration.

Well aware that I was not able to return to London, I decided to look for a contract working with indigenous women in remote or rural Australia. When I first decided to come to Australia, I focused on getting work close to Melbourne so I could spend time with my family. Now I would have to wait it out and could scratch the itch of returning to remote work - something I had wanted to do, but decided against because I would only be in Australia for a few months

I sat for hours renewing and updating competencies online: hand hygiene, aggression management, how to put out a fire, medication management, midwifery specific competencies including breastfeeding, CTG, and new-born life support. It was laborious, but I knew I wouldn't have to do it again. After this contract, surely the planes would be flying and I could get home.

Little did I know that by the end of the contract, the UK and Europe would be in a worse situation and heading into the winter months. I might need to get another contract.

And so, this became a recurring theme of my accidental stay in Australia.

When an agent called me on a Thursday to tell me Alice Springs had a position for a midwife, and yes, they could accommodate my "no night duty", and would also like me to cover some lactation consultancy shifts, I said yes.

6 STUCK IN AUSTRALIA

In my earlier life in New Zealand, when I was busy working and mothering, I had become a frequent watcher of travel shows. It was a great time filler when insomnia hit in the wee hours of the morning. I would snuggle under a blanket and whet my travel appetite. I earmarked two towns as must-see destinations. The first was Bologna in Italy, mainly because I learned that Spaghetti Bolognese, a frequent flyer on our family menu, did not actually exist. Fancy that? Authentic Bolognese sauce has no tomatoes in it! I also wanted to see the city's Fountain of Neptune which had four mermaids with water spouting out of their breasts. I've since used my own photo of the statue in breastfeeding presentations to colleagues.

The other place that caught my curiosity was Alice Springs. I remember seeing a brilliant blue-sky with a contrasting orange hill as a backdrop to a town centre that had colour and vibrancy. There were markets and flags flying, with indigenous art and people were smiling everywhere. A tangible invitation to explore.

So much happened in such a short time. I'd been going through the gruelling process of transferring my agency competencies to the

Rural and Remote team of Healthcare Australia and had been offered a contract to work in Kalgoorlie, a mining town 800 km east of Perth. Maybe it was a busy time, maybe it was the changes with Coronavirus and working remotely, but that particular agency seemed next to useless.

I was expected to start at Kalgoorlie on the Monday, but by the end of the day on the Thursday prior, no contract, travel arrangements, or information on my accommodation had been sent.

The agency was cross when I contacted them on Friday and they tried to intimidate me with a fine from the hospital. It was, however, their inability to understand that nurses and midwives need to know the details of contracts so they can plan their lives which was the issue. I learned from this experience that the agents are often young, have no idea what the difference between a midwife and a nurse is, and don't appreciate the stress of starting a new contract, in a new town, state or country. This was the beginning of the now necessary new structure "work from home." With closed borders both nationally and internationally, the nursing and midwifery agencies were in a flux.

Meanwhile, my agent Leigh, who had secured my Benalla contract, phoned me with news that there was a job in Alice Springs, and it would mean no night duty and included a role as a Lactation Consultant. I would need to go into quarantine for fourteen days which would be paid for, but I would not get any salary. I didn't know what quarantine meant, but as I had always wanted to work in Alice Springs, I said yes, on the spot.

Kalgoorlie would have to find another midwife.

The universe seemed to be looking out for me. I was going to Alice Springs.

"Be careful what you wish for." Or is it, "where the mind leads, the body follows," a philosophy that I subscribe to and teach in my hypno-birthing sessions. I felt incredibly excited and although I didn't have any real idea of what I was heading into, I felt intuitively that it would be an experience I would never regret.

Generous as always, my brother Peter said, "Are you going to drive to Alice? You can take the BMW!"

I toyed with the idea. To drive to Alice Springs was too good an opportunity to pass up, and I would have a vehicle to use while I was there. But it was an epic journey.

I decided to drive and tried not to overthink it. My brother's gentle nudge helped too.

It's fair to say that driving alone from Bunbury in Western Australia (WA) to Alice Springs in the Northern Territory (NT) is a bloody outstanding achievement. The distance is the equivalent of London to Egypt, but on my map, it was a simple route. East for a couple of days, then a turn left and head north, arriving in the middle of Australia's Simpson Desert.

I was nervous at the start. Reluctant even. I'd done what I considered a similar journey in 1979 as a young and independent teenager. I had fled the boredom of Invercargill, my hometown at the bottom of Aotearoa, New Zealand, and relocated to Taranaki on the North Island. It seemed a similar feat, yet in reality, that was only a quarter of the distance ahead of me now.

Back in 1979, I had purchased my first car. It was a 1963 Ford Prefect, with vacuum window wipers that were disastrously slow going uphill, my nose had to be almost stuck to the windscreen, in order to see where the road led. Then when going downhill, the wipers would become manic trying to wipe the rain off the window before it had time to leave the cloud. But all said, it was an uncomfortable but reliable wee car.

I was about to upgrade.

The 90's vintage BMW was such a bloke car. Apparently, a good buy, my brother Peter insisted; he had paid a few thousand for it just before the motor packed it in. Instead of scrapping it, he found a new engine and spent as much as he had paid in the first place.

"Are you sure you want to do this?" said the voice of reason in my head. "I've got this," I replied, hoping like hell I had.

I'd only come to Australia for six months, and now, instead of going home to London, I was going to the back of beyond.

The pandemic that was brewing held a shadow of uncertainty for many. I had to make the most of the opportunity that presented itself. After all, it would all blow over soon, I felt sure of it. I focused on what was right in front of me, and for yet another phase of my life, took it one day at a time.

My contract would be for four months, so I gathered my two suitcases, my endless and growing paperwork files, and domiciliary essentials. I had a lovely wicker basket with a pretty cereal bowl, spoon, tin of Weetbix, long-life milk, thermos, coffee plunger, and Illy coffee. In the boot, I had the equivalent of three litres of water per day, and I had two litres ready beside me for drinking.

I toyed with the idea of swag and sleeping on the side of the road, but I thought it a step too far on my wilderness excursion and decided to stay in roadhouses. I had a duvet and pillow on the back seat for emergency sleeping. I had the 12th edition of Australia road and 4WD, Hema's most detailed road atlas, and a phone holder so I could use Google maps.

I'd been told that there are alcohol restrictions and food is costly in the Northern Territory, so I stocked up on basic provisions, like Hennessy's Cognac Prosecco, Twining's English Breakfast Tea, and Wattie's Tomato Sauce. Ohh and Marmite.

I also ensured I knew how to check the oil, water, and tyre pressure, how the cruise control worked, and the trusty radio. I wondered if I would get radio reception. Would Google maps work? I would soon find out.

I knew I would need some help to change a tyre, so I ensured I knew where the jack was and how to access the spare.

The electric seat adjusted to my height and the mirrors were all set; the vehicle was ready.

I woke before my alarm the day I left, filled the thermos with coffee, and loaded the freezer packs into the chilly bin.

"Right, so I'm off," I announced to BB(big brother), the bravado disguising my anxious shallow breaths. I just needed to go.

My mind went back to the time I had bungee jumped off Kawarau bridge years earlier. After waiting and waiting for the double act in front of me, my anxiety built to such an extent that I leapt just after the countdown to five and before the instructor could say four.

The anticipation of the journey reminded me of that jump. I just needed to get on the road before I chickened out.

My odometer registered 327724, the red spike on the gas gauge pointed to F, and the tires were at 36 kpa! I adjusted and readjusted the seat, the steering wheel position, and the rear vision mirror, then backed out of the driveway.

A teary-eyed BB (big brother) waved goodbye to me. Tears dripped down my face as I wondered when I would see him again. Although we knew very little of how Coronavirus would affect us in Australia, my brother and sister had medical conditions that I felt could be compromised were I to go back and forth to work at the local hospital. Going remote seemed like a sensible option.

I cried until I got to the first intersection, about 30 seconds down the road, and the Satnav told me to go left; BB had told me to go right. Fuck!

I phoned BB. "Keep it simple sis, just follow your Satnav till you are on the main road".

That's exactly what my kids say too!

I stopped crying.

As the sun was rising over Bunbury, my journey began. For the first of many times, I shuffled my arse into the seat, pulled back my shoulders, and, checking all the mirrors, took a long slow deep breath.

My journey had begun.

When in London or travelling around Europe, I was often unsure which direction to take. My brain was like, *"Hell sister, you are on the wrong side of the road, and north is like over there, and turning left is north. Right. Got that? Yeah, no."* But as I drove, the sun was directly in my eye, so I knew I was travelling east, and east is it for the next three days at least.

The reassurance that my sense of direction was correct, lulled me.

7 KANGAROOS AT DAWN

Everybody keeps telling me this - look out for kangaroos at dawn. And they also feed at dusk – they tell me that too. I must be honest; if another person tells me to look out for the kangaroos on the side of the road during sunrise, I will jump on them with the force of a roo buck's hind legs.

I did keep watch, of course, though it was challenging when the sun was in my eyes, but either I didn't watch carefully enough, or they were not doing what they always do. I did not see one at dawn or dusk for the entire journey.

There were a couple on day two in the middle of the day, and I was like, WTF! Nobody told me about this hazard, kangaroos at lunchtime?! In my solitude, I found this amusing and it occupied my thoughts for the next few kilometres.

Along with warnings about spotting kangaroos that jump out in the middle of the highway, I was repeatedly told that the borders were closed and I would need paperwork in order to cross. I found it incredible that, as a midwife, people would think I might hop in a car and drive for five days across three states without knowing what I needed. Mostly I just smiled, though feigning shock and surprise was tempting.

These were the early days of border closures, so knowing what paperwork I needed was impossible to find out. I had some documents which included my passport, driver's licence, and my work contract in Alice Springs. Also proof of address for Bunbury, a letter from the hospital confirming my quarantine, and my Medicare card. Of course, I joined the RAC (Roadside Assist) even though I was forewarned that there is no cell phone reception in most parts of Australia outside the cities and main towns.

Am I allowed to say that the prospect of being stopped by police and crossing borders seemed a bit of a bonus? It might add some seasoning to the long journey? I hoped it wouldn't be as dramatic as the Serbia Hungary Border. Surely not, I mused. I could vividly recall that journey. The sluggish, aged train my youngest son, Vinny and I were travelling on had come to a halt, and we faced questioning from various authorities—our bags were scrutinised, and our passports confiscated - not once, but three times. Surprisingly this time, my journey through Australia unfolded with encounters involving guns, barbed wire, and a variety of authorities. I had naively anticipated a straightforward experience, only to sense a looming threat towards the journey's conclusion, reminiscent of the unease I had felt on that European journey. There had been guns and barbed wire fences separating those countries.

Here in Australia I was more prepared. I had stocked up with boxes of *Celebrations* (chocolates) to thank my fellow essential workers en route. They were dragged into this border closure chaos as much as I was.

Cop Stop #1

Border Patrol. My first stop was close to Darkan, at 7:30 am. Not only had WA closed its borders with the other states, but they had also placed travel distance restrictions, limiting residents to 150 km from their homes. This was going to be a long journey to the SA border. I had my supply of Belgian chocolates but it seemed far too early to be giving these out.

Mr. Plod waved me down and meandered over to my window. "Where are you off to? A little bit of shopping in town?" he said in a tone that would bore the pants off Fr. Stone (season 1, episode 2 of Father Ted).

He hadn't even said good morning!

I took a second or two to plan my reply and eventually said, "Nah, I'm going to Alice Springs." Then I followed that up with, "Don't suppose you expected that answer?"

I'll give him the benefit of the doubt and say he was probably at the end of his shift and just wanted to go home, but his eyebrow-raising was his nonverbal reply.

"Can I see your licence and paperwork?"

I extended my driver's licence and opened my rather large plastic container of "documents." Along with my work contract, I handed over the WA border pass and a wad of papers. He filled out forms, ticking boxes.

He was in no hurry.

Perhaps a little disappointed that he didn't question me more about the marathon journey ahead, I was allowed to drive away, the sun now out of eyeshot and kangaroos tucked up under the trees. Plenty of chocolate was still tucked away in the chilly bin too.

I'd be giving them to friendly cops, and he wasn't a great start in the friendly department.

I hadn't considered road workers to be essential services. In WA, there were a surprising amount, and plenty of people were working.

On the outskirts of a town near Gundaring, I had to stop. I was the only vehicle that was not part of the works; but stop I did. And waited. And waited some more. After an agonisingly long wait, out of the dust ahead, came a utility vehicle with flashing lights. It did a u-turn in front of me. The lady in her high viz jacket holding the sign flipped her board and gave an almost imperceptible nod as if we were in some conspiracy together. The utility vehicle drove off ahead of me, revealing a sign chained across its boot - FOLLOW ME – so I did. I obeyed the sign and followed it for a long distance, being careful to avoid the dust it kicked up. Eventually, I came to a stop when a utility vehicle with flashing lights turned off the road to the left. Fortunately, I realised that I needed to keep going straight ahead to where the paved road continued. Even though I was tempted to follow the utility vehicle and have a 'smoko' break and a light banter with them, I decided not to and continued on my way.

I was back on the tar seal, and my cruise control cranked back to the steady 110kph.

Cop Stop #2

A sign ahead declared, 'Travel restrictions are in place. Prepare to stop' pre-warning drivers just past the town of Coomalbidgup.

I tried to say this out loud, "*Coo am elbid jub jup.*" "*coom albid gup.*" but couldn't manage very well. My tongue just went into overdrive with a lalalalalllla. That was the first time I talked to myself on the trip. It happened again over the next few days. Singing, yelling, self-counselling, laughing, singing out of tune, and making up words. No one answered me or told me to stop. It was the best part of driving solo.

I was hoping that cop at stop #2 they would at least have something interesting to say. Ahead was a square white tent with two camp chairs strategically placed in the shade with a view along the road. The orange cones directed me towards the tent, where I pulled up and wound down the window.

A police car with E201 written back to front, and the words 'POLICE' right way up, was parked on the other side of the canvas. I've always been curious about why they don't have both the words 'police' and the number back to front so it can be recognised in the rearview mirror.

A tall officer stood up from the chair and flagged me down. His partner kept reading something, more captivated by the book than by my presence.

Different questions this time - different papers as well; but at least he had a vague interest in why I was going to Alice Springs.

"You've got a way to go then," he said, "why are you going to Alice Springs?" I can't remember what I said. I must have made it up as it was a question I couldn't answer. Yes, I had a job, but the answer was a lot more complex than this. Because of Covid? Because I was stuck in Australia? Because I needed to go somewhere? Perhaps it was just because. It seemed a long time ago that I had first seen this intriguing town on the telly, not for a minute then did I imagine I would be working in Alice Springs

Cop at stop #2 got my first box of chocolates. As it transpired, his partner was his wife, and he asked if he had to share. I said, *"they're not for sharing,"* and called out the window to the young woman, "those are for you."

He laughed, and I drove off.

Cop stop #3

Bob is a truck driver. I'd met his wife, Sue when I first worked in the outback in 2006. Facebook has its uses, and I messaged Sue. Bob gave me a travel plan that avoided the dirt roads and 'short cuts'- the vital stuff that Google maps doesn't know about and the map book didn't clearly define.

It sounded lovely. Through Wagin, where there is an enormous ewe as the town mascot, onto Lake Grace, Lake King, then Ravensthorpe, *where you will need to get fuel* Bob wrote, down through Esperance, then up to Norseman.

The tourism board wrote, *If you enjoy checking out all things 'big', you must visit the Giant Ram*

It was hard to miss and not something I needed to stop to look at. I could see the giant white ram from the comfort of my vehicle. I said,

"Gidday, Mr. Ram," as I tootled on through the town, knowing my next landmark was a lake.

Lake Grace wasn't the Lake Garda of Australia that my imagination had conjured up. The map book showed an expansive sizeable blue lake. Google maps - although offline - showed me as a blue dot driving along a straight road through scrolls of grey and white swirly patterns which I realised were dried salt beds. It was beautiful to see on my screen. Stolen glances as I traversed the bridges spanning the lake confirmed the expanse was mother nature's beauty in her raw state, an ever changing palette of random circles.

Aboriginal art?

When I arrived at Lake King, I looked forward to seeing more of nature's beauty. What I saw was a natural landscape with colours of grey taupe, white as snow, and rust and red edges on the straight roads that cut straight across the spectacular flat expanse.

Awe. Gratitude. Wonder. Space.

It was hard to keep my eyes on the road.

I stopped to breathe and look and then breathe some more.

Being present is easy when you are amongst wonders.

I took Bob's advice, filled up with petrol, planning a lunch break in Esperance. By this time, my bladder was singing loudly. There are clean and easy-to-find public facilities in Esperance.

Esperance was *cracking down on tourists*. I read about this the next day. That's why I was stopped again! Three in one day – cop stop #3 was just a flash of the licence, a couple of random questions, and I was waved on. The seaside town was sadly empty. The stillness gave the sea more voice, and the gulls were hovering silently, devoid of the tourist crumb.

I was heading to Norseman and happy not to chat with copper #3. I was thinking of those bloody kangaroos that might know it was coming to dusk.

8 NORSEMAN OR HORSEMAN

The intrigue of a town named after a horse, with camel sculptures as its mascot, called Norseman, was underwhelming. I checked into the somewhat dingy roadhouse motel, put my walking shoes on, and went to explore.

It was a no-contact check-in. I could phone my dinner order and collect from the restaurant which had the chairs stacked on the tables, clearly telling clients that there was no dining-in option.

I think the Kiwi/Oz term 'bogan'[1] must have originated in this WA town.

Outside the supermarket, (a potential place to buy some food for dinner), three bogans stopped their riveting conversation and didn't even try for discretion as they watched me walking towards their patch. The tallest of the trio, a man in jeans and a black tee shirt with an indecipherable animal with horns on the front, and a mullet reaching the shoulders along his lanky neck, took a long last drag on his cigarette and dropped the butt on the footpath. Without taking his eyes off me, he stubbed it out with his sandal-clad foot, clinging to what I imagined to be hairy toes. The other two didn't move, also somewhat riveted by my arrival. Thank God, I had my dark sunglasses on. Oh, was that what they were staring at? My Prada sunglasses. They are big, round, and have delightful curly arms. I must have looked as strange to them as they did to me.

Inside the supermarket, the weather-skinned middle-aged woman with body art on her ample cleavage smiled and said, "Gidday," as I entered. "Sing out if you need a hand, love."

She seemed nice, so I felt obliged to buy something. The prepared salads and prepackaged foods had a tired look; the fresh fruit had lost its shine and like the shop owners' skin was wrinkled from the moisture-sucking heat. I found a super-inflated box of English breakfast tea bags and a packet of ginger nuts.

"That's all, thanks," I said to the woman who was carefully cutting the tops off the NORSEMAN TODAY local paper with gigantic scissors.

She rang up the two items. "Nothing like a good dunking," she said as I tapped my card to pay. She was referring to the ginger nut biscuits, I realised, as I waved goodbye.

The lads were still outside. Still watching. Still silent. Their stare followed me across the road.

The liquor store had a bogan female on reception. Her chair was tipped into the reclining position, one leg was crossed over the other so her foot was resting on the countertop, providing a clear view up to her knicker line. The small space was filled with ceiling-to-floor boxed wine, bourbon, and slabs of beer. The single bottles of wine were limited in number and were cheap blended grape varieties. The girl continued to talk to her boyfriend rather than serve me, so I just left. I don't think she even noticed I had been and gone.

The constant bark of guard dogs accompanied me back to the respite of the now-not-so-dingy, roadhouse room.

I settled for in-room dining. The otherwise delicious, freshly cooked meal lost its appeal when dished onto polystyrene plates to be eaten with plastic cutlery.

I have a stunning shot of a closed-down shop in this bogan town. The wrought iron is painted a brilliant green, a veranda of red iron providing shade from the walls to the edge of the footpath. The Fair Dinkum Ozzie building.

Norseman had seen better days. I think I'll stick to that photo memory and not bother to go back to Norseman.

My first night on the road. I slept. I did not dream.

9 THE NULLARBOR

With the ever-looming threat of the kangaroos causing chaos, I calculated the dawn and sunrise and allowed time to decant the coffee into a thermos, ready to hit the road at 6 am. I had checked the map and was about to start on the infamous route.

The mere mention of the *Nullarbor* elicits a response from every Australian.

Like Route 66 in the USA, it has its own legend and mystique.

"I'd love to drive across the Nullarbor," or "Now that's a drive not to be taken lightly."

"It takes a few days across the Nullarbor." "You have to drive across the Nullarbor?" Disbelief rhetoric. "How many days to drive all that way?" or simply "Wow! The Nullarbor."

When I said, "BB(big brother), I'm going to take your car and drive to Alice Springs," his reply, of course, included a reference to the road. Encouragingly he stifled his angst and thoughtfully said, "You'll love the Nullarbor LS(little sister); it's a great road, and not many have travelled that one."

Even though I had studied the map, I hadn't anticipated how flat and straight it was. I'm talking REALLY flat and REALLY straight for 1674 km. I thought I might get bored. I assumed I'd get sleepy. Would I have enough audiobooks? Did I download my Spotify playlist?

The Nullarbor (Latin for 'no trees') is a limestone plain over 700 km wide, stretching between the towns of Norseman and Ceduna. At its widest point, it is about 1200 km. It's the main route from Western Australia to the Eastern States via Adelaide.

I had known of people who had "driven to Perth across the Nullarbor" and dismissed them as crazy, wondering why they would want to drive. Many choose to fly and send their cars via transporters.

I tried not to overthink it.

I discovered, on day two of my journey and day one of the Nullarbor, that cruise control is a driver's best friend. Each day, I would need to overtake 2-3 road trains; but other than adjusting my speed at such times, it was set at 110 km p/h.

I had downloaded the Podcast "My Father Wrote a Porno." This kept me giggling and reminded me of Teddy in my writers' group back in London. Teddy had been bending the unwritten rules of our Highgate set and had been infiltrating the Wednesday mornings with borderline porn. There had been a flurry in the writing group, and then he stopped coming. I flirted with the idea that maybe we should do a podcast of his stories. These guys had made a mint from very mediocre storylines.

Two days into my journey, my long-held belief that Australia was "a shit load of nothing" wasn't actually true.

Subtle changes in the colours and shrubs showed the perceived barrenness was alive and abundant. Even the colours of the tarmac roads changed with the land going from grey to red and back to desert tawny.

Void of landmarks, this road slithers through the subtle geology of its landscapes. I was infused with the sensation of insignificance against the backdrop of expansive terrain. On the road, it was as though I had this secret to myself. I felt welcome. I felt safe.

It was wonderful.

10 AUSTRALIA'S LONGEST STRAIGHTEST ROAD

There is a state of subconsciousness that the Nullabor lulls you into. Semi-hypnotic, the vista changes as the sun moves across the sky. There are few shadows, yet the shrubs and sandy dirt constantly change through autumnal shades. Crows eating the roadkill keep you alert. Easily seen in the distance as black blobs feasting on their tucker, it's best to slow down if it is safe. Their bellies full and their reactions slowed by their food coma, they take off at a staggeringly slow upward lift and turn away from the vehicle just in time, or so it seemed to me. I didn't see many dead crows, so maybe their ability to judge the speed was better than I imagined.

On a section of road with no roadkill in site, my brain was occupied listening to a podcast as I drove past the road sign heralding:

90 MILE STRAIGHT

AUSTRALIA'S LONGEST STRAIGHT ROAD 146.6km

But did I just see a man up a ladder against the sign? Or was I seeing things?

It was so strange; my brain couldn't fathom what was happening. I hadn't seen a vehicle let alone a human, all day.

I checked through the rearview mirror and confirmed it was a ladder and a person. There was also a white work vehicle parked under the sign that I had missed entirely.

I concluded that the man was replacing the sign. I'm sure it got nicked all the time, a prized trophy in sports bars or game rooms.

I'd be checking the bogans' pool room in Norseman if I were him.

This 90-mile section of road spans from Balladonia in the west to Caiguna in the east and is 90 miles straight, really straight.

There are roadhouses welcoming weary travellers every 200km. I'm sure they sell t-shirts and car stickers that confirm the 90 miles. I didn't stop, so I don't have a bumper sticker or t-shirt. Just the memory.

I later read that this straight road would have held the world record, but for a road in Saudi Arabia that is almost twice as long – but just as straight.

Just past the start of the 90-mile straightest road, there was another road sign with three diamond-shaped placards with a yellow background. The first was a black stencil of a camel distinguished with a hump and spindly dancing legs. The second was a blobby-looking animal with a very white eye, presumably a wombat. The last was a stunningly obvious kangaroo. These triangle depictions were attached to a sign that said NEXT 96km. I know it was a warning, but I was very excited that I might spot a wombat or a camel.

No camel. No wombat. No kangaroo, but of course, I knew they came out at dawn and dusk when I wouldn't be driving. A lone dingo did run out in front of me, a fair way in the distance. Lindy Chamberlain came to mind. There were also the graceful and beautiful hawks, whose distinctive feathers and tails fanned to catch the thermal, spiralling upwards and swooping down. Rather than high in the sky, the birds of prey kept low to the land. I'm not sure why. They, too, would partake in some of the truckie's leftovers.

Along every highway in Australia, there are rest stops, roadhouses, and viewpoints. Each state has its version of symbols to alert the traveller. On the Nullarbor, the viewpoint has a sign of a camera, picnic stops have a picnic table symbol, and they each will have guidance as to whether there is water, toilet facilities, if you can camp, and if you can leave your rubbish. All are designed to be deciphered in any language. The road trains have their own stops as they need a lengthier driveway and stopping distance. A car with a line through it is a no-go for a traveller.

I came to a viewpoint and pulled into the area. There were picnic tables for use, but the road to the whale-watching tourism venture was closed due to coronavirus.

The fresh air was a welcome and great relief to stretch my legs and straighten my back.

I walked down the small track to the edge of the cliff and soaked in the vista of the Great Australian Bight as she rehydrated my desert-driving eyes.

Three menacing crows shattered this contemplative moment, which scared the bejesus out of me. Their distinctive caw caw caw echoed threateningly.

I don't like crows. I don't like birds. I'd been attacked by a rooster when I was three, and the memory of being swooped by a magpie in Benalla still harboured an innate fear.

I threw the delicious juicy peach I was eating in one direction, hoping it would act as a decoy, then ran back to the safety of the car in the opposite direction.

I wished I hadn't stopped.

What's the time?

What time I reached the roadhouse at Border village is still a mystery to me. I either arrived at 3:15, 4:00, or 4:45.

I stood and stared at the three clocks, each with the arms pointing to differing numbers like in a financial institution that needs to know the close of trading.

These three clocks were behind the reception at the roadhouse in the middle of the Nullarbor, where I was booked to stay the night. My mobile hadn't adjusted automatically. Or had it? I was confused.

The woman behind the till smiled and said, "Who knew huh? I moved here last week, and it was the first time I'd heard about this time zone."

"It's 4 o'clock, but if you go for a 5-minute drive to look at the cliffs, it will be later."

Who knew that there is another time zone between Western Australia and South Australia?

This time zone is for a distance of 350 km, officially based on the quarter hour, not the half hour or the hour. The time in this time zone is set halfway between the South Australia time zone (ACST) and the Western Australia time zone (AWST). So, it is 45 minutes ahead of WA time and 45 minutes behind SA time. Since Western Australia doesn't observe DayLight Savings (DST), this time zone (ACWST) doesn't observe DST either. Tiredness and maths didn't mix. I asked what time the kitchen closed for dinner and instantly regretted the question. I readjusted my question, "I mean, how much longer is the kitchen open?"

"Oh, till seven on the middle clock. Too easy", she replied, ending her statement with a smile.

I did go for a drive across the time zone to see the cliffs and again get my fix of the wild coastline and infinite sea. When I returned, the car park at the roadhouse had been filled with police vehicles, white 4 x 4 Toyotas, utility vehicles, and road maintenance trucks. My silver BMW sedan looked alien.

After another freshly prepared polystyrene-presented dinner in my room, I stepped outside to where the night sky had effortlessly replaced the day. I walked to the back of the accommodation dongas[1] and was wrapped in silence and moonlight within a few metres.

Van Morrison whispered in my ear, "*It was a marvellous night for a moon dance.*"

The largest super moon of 2020 rose in the wilderness as a floating yellow disc, dwarfing the beloved Southern Cross that was visible, pointing due south, to Aotearoa, New Zealand... to my homeland.

The expanse of sky seemed close enough to touch. The stars twinkled.

Twinkle, twinkle, little star,
  How I wonder what you are!
   Up above the world so high,
   Like a diamond in the sky.

When the blazing sun is gone,
  When he nothing shines upon,
  Then you show your little light,
  Twinkle, twinkle, all the night.

Then the traveller in the dark
  Thanks you for your tiny spark,
  How could he see where to go,
  If you did not twinkle so?

In the dark blue sky you keep,
  Often through my curtains peep
  For you never shut your eye,
  Till the sun is in the sky.

As your bright and tiny spark
  Lights the traveller in the dark,
  Though I know not what you are,
  Twinkle, twinkle, little star.

. . .

Thank you, Jane Taylor.

The milky way, with infinite depth and drama, gently wrapped her arms around my shoulders that night.
    Welcome home, she spoke.
    I slept floating in a time warp sprinkled with stars and moon dust.
    I did not dream.

11 ROAD TRAIN

The sun was awake enough for me to leave at an indeterminate time; hence, not knowing when I would arrive at Kimba. According to my map book, the border village roadhouse where I had stayed was on the geographical border, but border patrol was a few hundred kilometres through the Nullarbor planes. As I've already described, the road was straight and continued to be so, but the trees eventually replaced the disquieting flatness.

I needed a comfort stop, and Murphy's Law states that there are no stops when you need to pee. With a bursting bladder, I finally spotted an off-road rest area. This would have to be a beside-the-car pee, which is inevitable during such a long journey. It necessitates a risk assessment for snakes. I had yet to come across a slithery reptile and was not keen to encounter one with my pants down. I drove in and around the parking space and eventually finding nothing that would provide camouflage, I parked facing the sea. My concentration was on the task at hand.

Ah, the relief. There was nothing to see, but a cage-topped rubbish bin lined with a black plastic bag, strikingly empty.

Not even a tree for shade at this stop.

Ready to hit the road again, I was overcome with a brief yet disconcerting moment. I was unsure which direction to go. Such flatness for eternity. No cars to note the direction of travel. No signs. Most of the stops are the same, randomly on either side of the road.

I thought of the Aboriginal mob. What incredible skill they had to survive and navigate this land?

Heading East with my podcast resumed, I realised that I had not seen a single car travelling in the same direction as me and perhaps one each day in the opposite direction. Even the road trains were rare, and I had not seen a caravan. I would catch up with a road train every 2-3 hours. The travel restrictions had hit hard and fast. Such a surreal time to be travelling across this vast land. I felt as though I had the Nullarbor to myself. I felt I had all of Australia to myself. At the time, I knew it was an experience that I had neither anticipated nor imagined, but the loneliness, the silence, the emptiness would never happen again. I felt an indescribable gratitude to mother nature for sharing this moment in history with me because as the rest of the planet was festering, I was drowning in awe.

It was majestical.

Majestical, my favourite word from the classic Kiwi film, *Hunt for the Wilderpeople* by Taika Waititi.

I thought about this word often during my journey.

BB's BMW had a great motor, and as the roads were so bloody straight, there was no pressure to speed in order to pass the road trains safely. I've since had the misfortune of travelling behind an occasional grey nomad. They are the retired couples who sell up, cash up, buy a caravan, and spend a year or two touring before settling somewhere sunny or close to grandchildren. I've developed a dislike for their discourtesy. They hog the road, and unlike the road train drivers, don't give you any indication if the road is clear ahead for you to pass. The road train truckers are great.

From a distance, the road train signs on their vehicle warn you that they are not just a truck and single trailer. When they notice you are stuck behind for any length of time, they will give you the flick of their indicator to advise that the road ahead is clear.

Often there are convoys of *oversized* vehicles chaperoned with flashing lights and warning signs. So far, I had only seen this oncoming and it was around mining sites. These were always oversized, and I needed to stop on the side of the road to let one pass. This one was transporting accommodation huts, a ginormous truck, and equipment required for the mining industry. These guys often travel through the night, so it's not too common an encounter.

Road trains have to travel at 100kph in Western Australia and South Australia.

The most memorable road train I encountered was on this journey. I had spotted it in the distance and eventually caught up to it, indicated and then proceeded to pass it. Initially, it felt as though I wasn't actually overtaking. It went on and on. It was unnerving. The road ahead was clear, but all I could think was, "Fuck, this is long." I took it steady but put my foot down and cruised to a speed that would accrue demerit points if the radar clocked it. Eventually, I completed the overtake, gave the driver a wave, and soon left him behind. Or so I thought.

I had crossed the border to South Australia early in the morning and was now at the quarantine and newly set up coronavirus border patrol. There was a different set of paperwork required altogether, which I had, but it was in my paperwork file. This was finally done and then it was on to biosecurity; these regulations had slipped my mind.

As I threw my fresh fruit stash into the special receptacle, quietly wishing I'd thrown all the peaches at the crows the day before, the yellow Kalari road train pulled into the stop.

"Oh fuck," I said far too loudly. The policewoman just glared at me.

I qualified my cuss. "I overtook that just up the road. I knew it was big, but it's huge, I blurted. Now I'll be behind it again."

This particular road train had a cab plus four carriages with more than 40 wheels on each side. It must have been more than 50 metres long

I excused myself from the quarantine and coronavirus interrogation. I took a photo, knowing or hoping I'd never see a road train this length again, then proceeded to answer all the usual questions, show my papers, and was issued with an Essential Traveller Notice authorised by the South Australia Police.

D.R. Baker-Twog SGT 26950 reassured me that that train was just going a few kilometres along the road to the mining site and not to worry. I gave her a box of chocolates, and I got to drive on to Kimba.

I had driven halfway across Australia.

12 HALFWAY ACROSS AUSTRALIA

Maybe it is. Maybe it isn't, but Kimba boasts to be "halfway across Australia". The sign at the edge of the town has a picture of two tin figures, a mixture of thunderbird puppets and Tinman from The Wizard of Oz set. Carved out of metal, they stand tall against desert land. I hadn't planned to come this far down into South Australia, until fellow Kiwi Jeff, my other trusted source of information for driving around this great continent explained that my planned shortcut from Wirrulla to Coober Pedy was a gravel road. I would need a 4x4 if I was to go that route. So here I was on my sensible tar-sealed road, adding a day's travel, but arriving intact in this pretty little town.

It may seem peculiar, but sometimes I forget that I am in Australia. I know I am stuck here by accident because of the pandemic, yet I know I'm not in London or Aotearoa New Zealand. Passing the welcome to Kimba sign, I was momentarily displaced and confused with what I was seeing. The town was adorned with a trumpeting of ANZAC day flags flying from each of the town's street lamps, each with a poppy and soldier. It suddenly dawned on me, I was actually in the middle of Australia and would not be in Belgium on April 25th with my New Zealand Pilgrimage Trust friends at Menin Gate nor at the Passchendaele fields as planned. It was sobering. I felt cheated. I felt stuck.

I was in the middle of fucking Australia instead.

There were a few shops open in this pretty little town, independently owned with trendy window dressings as I drove to my accommodation.

I was horrified to arrive at a ramshackle row of concrete rooms and a wizened old man sitting fagging away outside.

Maybe I had got the wrong address?

I phoned the Airbnb host and was frosty with her, exclaiming it didn't seem an appropriate place for me to stay. Patiently Margaret, the Airbnb owner listened and offered to let me stay at another place, but suggested I first look inside and if I wasn't happy, she would change the room.

I finally agreed to at least have a look inside before being relocated.

I mentioned the old fella outside. She reassured me that Mick was a long-termer and would look out for me. This didn't reassure me as I took a sideways glance at the man who sat with his skinny legs plaited rather than crossed, sucking the life out of a rollie and sipping on his coffee mug.

Opening the apartment, I was treated to a flashback to the 1970s. The front lounge had an orange and brown circular carpet and a couple of two-seater vinyl sofas with crochet pillows in similar tones of brown. The sideboard was filled with crystal glasses, Wedgwood plates upright on little stands, a stack of Spode dishes and some green Limoges. In the bedroom, immediately to the left, were two single beds with candlewick bedspreads and fairy-down quilts folded at the end. Between both were a table and a touch lamp sitting on a doiley with pretty lace edging. There was a built-in dressing table and where I knew should sit a vanity set, was a large Spode vase that had a crack repaired and discretely turned to not show the obvious brown fault line. Through to the kitchen, the first thing I saw was a stainless-steel sink that had three taps in a row all Classic style wall top assemblies with cross handle design without any H or C to indicate their rank.

I forgot to find out why there were three taps over that sink. It was rather curious but not particularly out of the ordinary in this extraordinary wee house.

The galley kitchen was clean and well-stocked with pantry basics. There was no microwave, which dated the décor to the mid 80s.

In the fridge, there was a welcome pack with milk, butter and half a dozen eggs. By the jug were a plethora of tea and a packet of ginger nut biscuits.

I was charmed by this quaint accommodation. I thought of my mother.

I phoned Margaret back and thanked her for her patience. Yes, I would be happy to stay here.

At the local shop, I found a mini Prosecco which I enjoyed out of a Darlington glass champagne flute with gold filigree edging. There were leftover Easter eggs for sale. It was then I realised it was Easter weekend. For the second time in Kimba, I felt discombobulated.

I bought Mick an Easter egg. I apologised that it was an egg and perhaps should have been a hot cross bun as it was Good Friday. He smiled and thanked me in his slow Australian drawl; then with his rollie firmly held between two nicotine orange fingers pointed the way I could drive out the next morning to save having to turn around outside his house. He then re-plaited his legs, flicked the ash into the overfull tin can that he was using as an ashtray and assumed his stance as I had seen upon my arrival.

I realised it was not coffee he was drinking.

13 PRISCILLA QUEEN OF THE DESERT

Turning left couldn't come soon enough. I had joked with my brother that I probably wouldn't need a Satnav or Google maps? I'd just head towards the sunrise for a few days, then turn left. When this happened, I would dust off my Priscilla soundtrack and know I was getting closer to my destination.

I had a schoolgirl giggle at the signpost to Iron Nob wondering how it got that name.

The reality of what I saw after I left the eastern highway at port Augusta was distasteful. I felt uneasy and wasn't sure why.

For miles and endless miles were dirt piles like mini pyramids, trucks, tents, barriers on the roads and fences. I wondered if I was near the British nuclear testing area. A Google check confirmed I had been bordering the Maralinga site through the Nullarbor and now up to Coober Pedy.

Maralinga Tjartja land was the site of the British Nuclear Test Program between 1953 and 1963. About 1,200 Aboriginal people were exposed to radiation during the testing. The radioactive fallout, called "puyu" (black mist) by Aboriginal people, caused sore eyes, skin rashes, diarrhoea, vomiting, fever and the early death of entire families. The explosion had also caused blindness. This added to the displacement of the traditional owners. The land, now returned to its owners, is reported to be a vibrant cultural centre.

With *Priscilla* blasting from my speakers, I tried not to think of the land being raped, of people's plight and the innocence of the servicemen who worked there; but that was impossible.

There were rural myths of how people 'went missing' around this area. There were warning signs of a shaft and a person slipping down a hole to act as a deterrent to anyone thinking of climbing over the fences.

I've never liked opal. I now know why.

Coober Pedy was red, dusty, rocky and closed. I got a message from a colleague "you must get a Johns pizza! They are the best in Australia." It was the best thing about Coober Pedy. Thank god John sold beer.

I needed one that night.

Cattle graze freely through the desert and there are signs on the roadside to warn drivers where they are commonly seen. The signs are of course a caricature of a cow! I loved seeing the big beefy beasts along the highway and the wild brumbies. Thus far, I had only seen camels in the farms. I think I would have had to stop and photograph them had they crossed my path. Apparently, camels are now being exported to Saudi. That's a bit of a surprise, isn't it?

My animal spotting tally to date is along with a kangaroo, emu, a dingo and an echidna. There was a weird-looking bird that after some detective work was designated as a bush turkey. The aboriginal mob love them for tucker (food).

I hadn't heard of the Ghan until very recently. I spotted it on the travel channel. Think pre Covid-Michael Portello *Downunder* series, travelling on the Ghan. Like the Nullarbor most Ozzie's know about it. This iconic train travels the longest north-south train journey in the world. From Adelaide to Darwin. It must go through Alice Springs, I realised.

But like most Ozzies I don't think they know there is a town called Ghan?

This was for me Copstop #4. Or was it 4? I was losing count.

I was now in the Northern Territory (NT)and along with warnings of kangaroo behaviour and documents was warned to watch out for the NT police!

Their border patrol was strategically placed at the intersection with a minor road that had a lonely shell of "the old Ghan train" as a tourist attraction. That and flies were all that was there until the NT lockdown.

Mr Plod at Copstop #4 was a plainclothes detective. He gave me his business card. "Bet you are loving this job," I quipped. He smiled and rolled his eyes. I understood.

The set-up in the middle of nowhere had the usual bright cones, camping seats and shade for the Covid team. This one had the police Ute with the community engagement set up with a trailer and generator stretching up into the sky providing lights. The Police vehicles here were an unorthodox gold, with blue and white chequered sides and red and blue lights across the roof. Very American I thought. One thing for sure on this journey - I had seen my fair share of police cars, all of which were unique.

It took ages at this stop. I had to email my documents to Mr Plainclothes Detective, and he ducked in and out of his donga to confirm their safe passage to his laptop. I thanked him and gave him a taste of Belgium.

NT coppers were ok, I thought. I knew they had me on their books. My car and my documents were recorded.

Alice Springs was tantalisingly close.

I had made it through the border and passed an old Ghan train carcass.

It looked sad. Nearly there.

I settled into the last couple of hours without music, podcasts or audiobooks. I passed the turnoff to Uluru National Park. Realising I was so close to Uluru, thrilled me.

The haunting memory of little Azaria Chamberlain[1] and her mother's cry "a dingo's got my baby" seemed eerily present. Even though it was over forty years ago. In relative silence, I listened to my soul and drank in the isolation and privilege that this journey had offered. I knew I was one of a few to have travelled this road combining its geographical uniqueness and aloneness that the Covid 19 pandemic had afforded me.

I had driven 3000 kilometres with the highway to myself. I thanked the universe that I was spared the company of the grey nomads most of the way. The privilege of empty rest stops where I could pee if I had to was nice. I only had to worry about which way the direction the pee-stream would snake - typically, of course, towards my shoe. I could drive in the middle of the highway if I needed to or gawk at the scenery. I could slow down to watch or speed away as the crows were fed on the roadkill, and knew I wouldn't get rammed up the rear. All the towns were closed, and the services were quiet; this added to the magnitude of what was unfolding around the world.

Gratitude was foremost in my thoughts.

"I'm envious of you mum," said my youngest son from the flat in Highgate. "We are stuck here, and you are free to drive around Australia on an amazing adventure".

It was very grounding to hear.

Happy in my own thoughts for the final leg of the journey I soaked in the changing landscape and marvelled at the redness of the country.

Then a large and rather zany looking billboard advertising "The Thirsty Camel" caught my attention. Along with the camel licking its lips was a picture of tempting cool beer guaranteed to quell any desert thirst.

It was not my usual style to be brainwashed by billboards, but on this journey and on this, my last day driving across Australia, the thought of a cold beer caught me. The more I thought about it the more I was annoyed that in my pre-planning I hadn't actually thought of beer. I had Central Otago Pinot Noir, NZ Riesling and Hennessys tucked (and hidden) in the boot; but no beer. There was only one thing to do and that was to buy a six pack before I arrived in Alice even though I had strict instructions to drive directly to the quarantine facility.

Just beyond the first Thirsty Camel billboard was a roadhouse where I parked under the shady trees. The car park was empty, but the shop was open.

"Do you sell beer?" I asked the weathered man behind the counter. Disinterested and barely taking his eyes off the floor, he said "no".

"Oh, do you know where I can get some, then?"

"Just up the road might sell it."

Feeling a little guilty and sad that there were no customers, I bought a coffee which I discarded after one sip. I needn't have bothered but wondered how these roadhouses would actually survive these strange times.

Stanley Wells a further 100 kilometres.

Fully optimistic and back onto the Stuart Highway I felt weary but excited to be close to the journey's end.

Four more Thirsty Camel billboards promising the cool liquid, and two more roadhouse stops proved fruitless. "Only on tap" said the barman at the first stop and "we no sell take away alcohol" said the Thai cook at Stanley Wells Camel farm.

I gave up imagining drinking a cool beer and tutted myself for getting lured in by a billboard.

Another cop stop!

I was itching to get to Alice Springs. I had by this time lost count of how many times I had to prove who I was, show my contract details, answer random questions and justify my being on the road; so within 50km of what I thought would have been the last Covid patrol was another.

I had run out of chocolates. I had run out of patience. I had run out of nice.

I answered in monosyllables. I had the fist full of documents that I had ordinarily given selectively but shoved the whole lot into the policeman's hand.

His attitude matched mine. He scanned the first two pages and thrust them back to me.

That's all good, he said as he ticked a page on his clipboard.

As I prepared to leave I heard a grating grinding mechanical whirr. The electrics closed the window for the last time.

I finally turned left and ahead of me was the "Welcome to Alice Springs" rock I had seen on the postcards. I let out a spontaneous woohoo that cut the silence in the car.

I pulled in for a selfie and fired it off to Wellington, Cambridge UK Melbourne and London sending Aloha around the world to my children. Then I cried. In my heart I had always wanted to come to Alice, to work with the Aboriginal women. Although I was here somewhat by accident, the universe was looking out for me. I held on to this convolution of thoughts and feelings leaving them to rest. It was a changing world.

At the rock, I met the desert flies. These little beasts, black persistent and happy to stick to my skin and crawl into my nose and ears, arrived in great numbers. I didn't linger and had to wipe them off my clothing like a bad dose of dandruff before hopping back into the car.

The road into Alice meanders through a narrowing, which locals refer to as the gap.

The Heavitree Gap, or Ntaripe in the Arrernte language, is a gap in the MacDonnell Ranges of Central Australia.

It is the entrance to the city of Alice Springs and in addition to the Todd River it carries the main road and rail access to the South. The Gap was and still is a most important sacred site for the Arrernte people of the area.

Beyond this narrowing in the road is a roundabout that has two exits to the town centre. To the right, I could see not only the goofy looking camel but an actual Thirsty Camel bottle store.

As the cars peeled off to the bottle-o I made the split-second decision to divert and pick up a six pack of beer via a contactless drive-through. I would then set my Sat Nav for Palm Springs Resort.

Perfect!

As I pulled into the queue on the drive they came out.

Like the flies at the Welcome to Alice rock, the Northern Territory Police appeared out of nowhere. In slow motion. Four police officers, all with dark uniforms and wearing caps, emerged from under the drive through. Guns and batons hanging off their belts. I felt sick.

FUCK I said out loud. Busted! Fuck!

"Watch out for the NT cops," " go straight to your accommodation" " you can only stop for petrol" played across my mind. I bloody knew I shouldn't have chanced this...I wasn't that desperate for beer.

As a short cop who looked about ten years old came towards me, my guilt was a heavy weight.

His colleague a few paces behind was glaring at the WA car plates and tapping his mobile device.

He indicated he wanted to talk to me, but to add to the scenario playing out in slow-motion, the BMW window electrics had packed up and so I went to open the door.

The babyface cop instantly reached for his gun and took a step back. He stopped short of grabbing his pistol and put his hand up facing me to stop me opening the door. I mimed like a muppet that the window didn't work. He walked around the back of the car to the passenger side, poised ready to fire his gun.

Well, that's how it felt.

At the exit of the drive-thru, I noticed two other police officers who looked like they were ready to appear in a TV show, with the typical "I'm a police officer and I'm watching this" demeanour. Normally, I would have found it amusing or exciting, but at that moment my heart was pounding with anxiety. All I could think about was the headline that would follow: "Midwife arrested at Thirsty Camel drive-thru.

"Are you from out of state ma'm?" "Yes." I said with a smile.

"Where have you come from?"

"Um.. you mean today or..?"

"Where do you normally live?" he barked.

This was not an easy question to answer. I almost said London but thought that might spin him, so I said "Well Melbourne, but I've come from Perth"

"So why are you not in quarantine?"

I lied – sort of. "Oh, I'm on my way. I have quarantine when I get to Alice Springs. I have two weeks and I thought I would need beer" I said with a hint of a smile.

"You ARE in Alice Springs" he said incredulously.

"Really? my Sat Nav says I have ten kilometres to go." I lied again.

I had to keep my cool and get out of there without being thrown in prison or fined. The NT cops did have this reputation. I didn't think I'd have to worry. But now I was.

Babyface cop called his boss over. He was a tall Indian cop broad-shouldered and a don't-fuck-with me look on his face. One of the officers from the exit stakeout stood about three metres behind him. I could feel my heart thumping and knew I had to keep calm. I didn't realise I was in Alice's rhetoric.

Eventually, after taking my name and details, questioning my why I came here knowing I could put the community at risk while I was acting dumb, he said, "I'll have to decline your access to this facility. Turn around there, pointing to the back of the bottle-o and go straight to the accommodation."

I no longer needed a beer. I think I needed a stiffer drink.

I got the feeling baby cop really wanted to fine me but I knew I wasn't really breaking quarantine as I hadn't actually gone into it as yet.

This was the very early days of Covid cross border travel.

By now I was annoyed with the heavy-handed management. No longer feeling like I was going to be shot at and relieved to be let go, my defiant streak emerged.

"I need to get petrol, where is the closest station?" I wanted to prove that not allowing me to buy beer was a pointless decision.

Three police officers stood in a huddle discussing this question and maybe what to do with me. Babyface who by now was in charge of communicating with me through the passenger side window said, "you are allowed to get petrol."

I didn't say "I knew that you big galagh" but wanted to. It was a quiet win for me.

I closed the window, drove ceremoniously past the cars all lined up watching the mini drama unfold, then turned and went to the closest petrol station. I was shaken.

I set the Sat Nav to the safety of my quarantine unit. I arrived. Almost unscathed.

My speedo clocked 331627. 3903km or 2425 miles after leaving the security of my family in Bunbury.

There was a sign directing me to the unit. I was not to stop nor report into reception. I drove past identical units. Stress and anxiety and relief blanked any peripheral awareness.

Chalet Number 16 had two beautiful palm trees out the front that looked like tall pineapples. I parked outside and stepped onto the veranda where there was a glass top table and three plastic chairs. I looked around to where a bird's caw caw was coming from. To my right in the distance there was the red rock that I thought I may have passed on the way into town. The endless identical chalets had a towel or hammock set one off as different to another. The unlocked ranch slider opened into a tidy and modern bedsit including a small kitchenette wet room and toilet. Returning to the deck, I looked across the road to the barren slightly elevated desert soil with a barbed wire fence separating the holiday resort from whatever this land held beyond.

I visually mapped out my parameters. I realised that during my fourteen days of isolation ahead, I could either focus on the barbed wire fence or on the pineapple palms.

As it happened, there were days of both.

14 QUARANTINE IN ALICE SPRINGS

I hadn't imagined what two weeks of quarantine would be like. My limited awareness of quarantine was from school reading about islands in New Zealand for lepers' or a facility used to quarantine returned soldiers suspected of carrying influenza in 1919. It was a historical concept that seemed distinctly out of place in 2020. But here I was in Alice Springs, the middle of Australia, in a quarantine facility.

Or was it a resort? The self-contained chalet at Desert Springs was a single-room kitchen and bedroom, with a queen and single bed. The dining area was outside on the deck which I was allowed to use but not go beyond. There was a bathroom. I unpacked my worldly possessions, re-jigged the furniture, converted the single bed into a chaise lounge, draped my pashminas and jewellery over the tourist artwork and felt quietly optimistic that this would do nicely. There have been many times in my life that I craved the peaceful serenity of a resort in the sun, with nothing to do but write or read and was reminded of the mantra I teach in hypno-birthing, *where the mind leads, the body follows.*

Well, here I was.

With all the time in the world over the next two weeks, I had successfully occupied two hours.

Now, what will I do, I thought. The rollercoaster of emotions unleashed.

The Alice Springs hospital staff contact number I had been given was for "any queries or shopping needs during your stay, and for overall support." So I contacted Rachel and asked her to buy me some A3 coloured cardboard and felt tip pens.

"No worries."

"Oh and some beer? Can I buy beer?"

"Of course," she replied. She exchanged bank details and within the hour I had talked to the first normal person since the police encounter earlier which still rattled me.

As was the policy, Rachel would have to ask me to stay inside while she delivered the shopping onto the deck, and then she would step back. We were allowed to have a yarn[1] from a distance. She was young and energetic, apologising for buying a slab of beer but it was better value than the twelve pack and she laughed as she said, "most people just buy a slab, especially when they are in quarantine."

I told her my bottle-o story. She at first showed concern but then we both just laughed. "You'll soon get used to the cops here; some are alright, but there are some real tossers."

My first evening, from the relative comfort of my chalet, between television and the internet, I watched my friends and family in Europe and London become engulfed in the pandemic.

I really had nothing to be stressed about.

Day 2 Quarantine I wrote, *Be kind to yourself.*

I used my coloured paper and pens to draw up a list of my support crew around the world, separating them into time zones and sorting the time differences. I somehow felt that I might need to keep in touch. It was very reassuring to start with my family and friends in New Zealand, separating out the North island and South island, East coast and West coast, Australia, Malaysia, Slovinia, Romania, Latvia, Italy, Belgium, France, United Kingdom, Ireland, East and West coast America and Canada. Every timezone was covered! Any time of the night or day, someone would be there for a chat. This made me feel good.

I realised it was Easter Sunday. I had been given a Humpty Dumpty easter egg with irresistible beanies inside - so the packaging said. It had survived the trip across the Nullarbor but didn't see out the two weeks of quarantine.

One of my Italian friends had messaged to give me the heads up that Andrea Bocelli was to give a solo performance representing a message of love, healing, and hope to Italy and the world.

I watched the live stream with a heavy heart and with such incredulity seeing Milano empty. During the performance, the cameras switched to other main cities of the world, and I saw Trafalgar Square in a way I could never have imagined; then, the drone footage captured my neighbourhood shopping area of Crouch End. Barren of all that is vital to a city, the clock tower stood marking time. I was shocked and cried that deep, ugly cry that encompasses more than can ever be articulated.

It was heartbreaking.

I felt very isolated, alone, and desperately homesick. I phoned my son.

"Mum," he said, "you can't have a meltdown yet, it's only day three. You need to wait until at least next week." Words of wisdom from lockdown in Melbourne.

Somehow this made me smile, and I felt better immediately.

The early days were spent resorting, sleeping, writing postcards, and mentally adjusting to having to stay in Australia.

Air New Zealand sent me a computer-generated email reminding me to check into my flight to Sydney tomorrow! Stabbing reminders of how life had taken a swift turn.

'We are all in it together' became a catch cry as Zoom meetings had to be scheduled into my day. My global map with names of friends around the world and their various time zones: there would always be someone to call. YouTube was filled with free and accessible pilates or yoga. I tapped into my cultural group in London, Ngati Ranana who initiated a hundi club that set the challenge to do 100 press up/sit up/step ups each day as a fun accountability group.

I had midwifery competencies and work forms to complete, and although they seemed to take much longer than usual, I got them done.

I lost track of the day and date. I had no alarm. Everything seemed to take a long time to achieve.

It was surprisingly restful. I slept with the curtains open and each morning I would watch the sun rising over a red hill.

One day I had a visitor.

Not in the way we usually know visitors. He was an old, weathered-looking bloke with a Santa Claus beard and lanky hair.

He came to replace a broken chalet number next door. Neither his accent nor his look was Australian.

He was from Treviso. "Buono sera," I said. "Buono sera, come sta?" he obligingly replied, to which I responded, "Molto bene."

My entire Italian vocabulary was spent.

We chatted about Prosecco because Treviso is the home of Prosecco, and I felt it was important that he knew I knew this about Italy.

He chatted as he hammered number 17 on the door. Then he left.

A chance encounter that filled three minutes of my quarantine.

Two weeks passed.

I had calculated my journey from WA to Alice Springs, hoping that there would be no delays in starting the 14-day quarantine so I would be released by Anzac Day, 2020. Had the pandemic not hit the world, I would have been in Ypres, Belgium, for the dawn ceremony at Polygon Woods.

My quarantine time had been relatively unchecked. I was never visited or phoned; there were no locks on the gates. However, I stayed completely compliant and calculated my release date to be Saturday, 25th. I was so very excited.

My New Zealand Pilgrimage Trust colleagues would not be at

Ypres either. It was a poignant reminder of the desolate isolation the young soldiers would have felt. I imagined their homesickness and uncertainty was far worse than our plight at the beginning of this pandemic.

Anzac dawn service in Alice Springs had been cancelled. I decided I would have my own dawn ceremony on Anzac hill and set my alarm for the first time in two weeks. I was up well before dawn and made my way up Anzac Hill. The poignant taste of freedom needed to be celebrated. I was not alone in my desire to pay my respects in these unusual times. An artist had sculpted a metal banner with soldiers and the rising Australian sun. He had hired a truck and erected the piece facing East West. There was a scattering of uniformed army or territory personnel. Stragglers by themselves or in pairs stood apart from others. A loudspeaker system was tuned into the Darwin Dawn service broadcast.

I believe it was the most magnificent showcase of mother nature's sunrise that I had ever encountered. The sun shone through the metal artwork, and the golden rays reflected off the red ranges as those of us gathered reflected upon our own personal thoughts as we listened to the broadcast. I sang with pride the NZ national anthem and the few words I knew of the Australian anthem.

As I write this, I am prompted to recall my first Australian Anzac day back in 2007 while I was working a morning midwifery shift in Northam, a town about 200k from Perth. In this quiet rural hospital was an elderly gentleman I cared for. As it happened, he had the telly on, and the Anzac commemorations were his main channel of interest. I sat on his bed, watching as the New Zealand anthem was performed. I sang along very casually, and back then, I didn't know the words in Te Reo Maori.

I joined in with my patient as he sang the Ozzie one.

Chatting with him, I said, "It's the spirit of Anzac, isn't it... a Kiwi and an Ozzie in the same room, both singing each other's anthems. "It is what it's all about, isn't it?"

"Do you know where I'm from?"

I didn't.

"Austria," he said.

"Oh, I've never been to Austria," I pondered.

Although I had been living in Ireland, I had not travelled in Europe at this stage, and my geography was rather limited. He seemed distracted and looked me in the eyes and said, "I was with the SS."

Perhaps the incongruity of the time and place or the disbelief and confusion made me silent. The SS? What is he talking about? Surely not the Nazis?

Ridiculously I thought about *The Sound of Music* remembering it was filmed in Salzburg, Austria. It took some time for me to speak. Until I asked a simple question.

"Did you know what you were doing back then?"

In all honesty, I assumed the answer would be, "Of course we didn't – we were young, and we were doing what everyone else was doing. No one knew what was happening." But to my surprise, he hung his head and answered, "Yes, we knew what we were doing."

I remember this anecdote each Anzac day. Without judgement or debate. It was my first personal insight into the human side of war.

Back in Alice Springs, after the sun was high in the sky, I got a coffee from the drive-through burger joint and found my way to my accommodation. It was in one of two three-story brick accommodation blocks within the hospital compound. My room was on the ground floor, number 37. I opened the door to a room identical to my first-year nursing days in New Plymouth in 1980. Single bed, study desk with chair, and another lounge chair. Double full-length wardrobe, a hand basin, and mirror.

Thirty years on, and this is what I had come to. I cried.

15 MPARNTWE, ALICE SPRINGS

The Aboriginal name for Alice Springs is *Mparntwe* (pronounced mm-BARN-doo- uh) but I have met very few non-indigenous people who knew this, even though it has been called this for tens of thousands of years.

Charles Todd, originally born in Islington, the suburb just down the road from my London flat, was a pioneer who orchestrated the single-wire connection from Adelaide to the rest of Australia, through Darwin and eventually with England in 1872.

It was one of the greatest engineering achievements of the nineteenth century.

The telegraph track followed that of another pioneer John Stuart; however, they needed to deviate through the Macdonnell Ranges. In 1871, the Simpsons Gap and the newly named Todd River, which was a vast dry riverbed with numerous water holes and springs, were discovered.

The principal spring was named after his wife, Alice.

I was curious to explore the town bang smack in the middle of Australia, central to Adelaide in the south and Darwin to the north. I wanted to get to know the community and see what the town was like.

It appeared steeped in history but was more famous for the surrounding Arrernte lands and the gorges and springs. It is the base camp for exploring Uluru and Kings Canyon, 400-500km southwest.

16 MIDWIFERY IN ALICE - AN ETHICAL DILEMMA

Alice Springs was surprisingly different from what I had expected. The maternity ward is set amidst the main hospital that seemed to be staffed by a young cohort backed up by people who notoriously came for a year and forgot to go home.

There was a medical model of care headed by opinionated and passionate obstetricians. The core midwives - many of whom had a strong midwifery passion and care for the women - had either succumbed to giving up fighting for a midwifery model or had managed to secure creative ways around it, depending on which consultant was about.

Perhaps this was the seed of discontent I felt permeating the unit. Everyone was watching everyone else, professionally and privately. There were overt cliques.

Like many rural and remote hospitals, being an agency midwife is not a novel concept, and I was just a name on a roster with no allowances made for being new. When I arrived, I waded my way through the new systems and protocols, relying on the tolerance of colleagues.

I found it incredibly difficult to know who was who, as the

students were allocated a patient load, new graduates were put in charge, and the skill mix was only considered if there were enough to cover the roster. We wore whatever we wanted. Officially, there may have been a uniform.

Alice Springs is the referral hospital for women in the Northern Territory beyond Tennant Creek, to the north, and the many communities in the great deserts surrounding. Women arrive in town two weeks before the baby is due and stay until transport back to their communities can be arranged once the baby is born.

Having a baby is an uncertain time for them. I'm unsure if they survive it unscathed.

Australia grapples with a persistent issue that perplexes me—the pervasive inequality among indigenous Australians, Torres Strait Islanders, and those from the Western culture. While the country endeavours to bridge this gap, my concern centres on the disparities across various levels. Despite substantial investments in schemes and rebranding services, a simple, cost-effective change in the childbirth policy could initiate positive transformations for the next generation.

Currently, except for a handful of isolated communities that have embraced "birthing on country" services, first-time mothers receive funding for a support person during childbirth and their hospital stay. However, with the arrival of their second child, this support is no longer funded. Consequently, these mothers are expected to navigate the birthing process alone, or rely on personal funds from their support person, partner, or other family members.

This system, imposing barriers on women, appears unique among civilised nations. Not only are they restricted from birthing on their ancestral land, but they are also unable to bring the comfort of their culture or support with them. In conversations with every woman I engage with, a common theme emerges—pain and disappointment. Some critics argue that these women receive sufficient government assistance and should cover their own expenses for childbirth, displaying a level of ignorance that seems insurmountable.

I propose a different vision—one where we actively support

women during pregnancy, addressing their holistic health, preventing ailments like anaemia and treating STDs. Encouraging a lifestyle free from alcohol, promoting a healthy diet, and providing a culturally safe birthing environment could be the initial steps to break the cycle of self-destruction.

However, I emphasise that this change must come from the women themselves. I convey to them, "As a white individual, my voice holds little relevance. Your voice is the one they will heed."

Across most states, in Australia, it is the same. It is called 'sit-down'. Non-indigenous women can choose to give birth in the local hospital, though many will go to a major city for 2-3 weeks prior to the birth and stay with family.

Postnatal care is universal. I noted early on in Alice Springs that the indigenous women shared a room and the non-indigenous women had single rooms. This may seem inequitable; however, I've learned that young Aboriginal women don't like being on their own in hospitals. Current pandemic rules that were still evolving, exacerbated this isolation for many. Hospital rooms can be hostile, lonely places. I've been asked many times by indigenous women to be moved to a different room or to keep a door open. They sense ghosts. They counter this by picking up their babies and going for a walk outside, downtown, or to the park. They return having had a feed from one of the fast food outlets. Many will buy a pram if the shops are open, but others just hold the baby in their arms. They would sleep till late. Breakfast was not a joyful meal, so it was mostly left untouched.

As indicated by the recruitment agent, I'd had my hopes set on working as a Lactation Consultant. It proved to be an awkward arrangement for reasons I could not actually figure out. For two allocated shifts, I would "help out in the lactation clinic." To help is patronising, but it was a means by which the organisation would not need to pay me the specialist rates.

The clinic operated out of the midwifery group practice (MGP) facility at the back of the hospital. This handful of strong independent midwives who I think were considered 'them' ('us' being the hospital-based team), were kind, supportive, interesting, and motivated.

My practice, and knowledge base was mostly congruent with the lead LC (Lactation Consultant), who had followed in the footsteps of two strong-minded LCs who had set up the service; both had recently retired.

I tried to be professional, kind, and engaging, but it was challenging at times.

I had professional expertise in addressing infant feeding issues related to a condition in a baby's mouth called "tongue tie." However, I found myself at odds with certain ethical aspects of the current practices in Alice Springs. As I shared my management preferences, my colleagues began to express their own concerns about what had become a normal practice in their community.

I discussed my concerns directly with the LC, who, in my opinion, had perfected a passive-aggressive response.

During an education session to the midwifery team, I shared the current evidence on ankyloglossia and oral frena, which was presented in the recently published Ankyloglossia and Oral Frena Consensus Statement by the Australian Dental Association and adopted in New Zealand. Although the guidance was consistent with my clinical expertise, it also pointed out that some local practices were outdated.

Perhaps opening my mouth was my undoing, but I was not offered an extension to this contract. Besides, they were waiting for the position to be filled by one of the core midwife's friends, a colleague of hers who sounded like the goddess of midwifery. I could never compete.

***

She was stuck in New Zealand. I thought of the irony. I was stuck in Alice Springs.

Oh, the places you'll go and the people you'll meet. Dr. Seuss must have been to the desert.

So now, I find myself by accident in the middle of what is euphemistically named the Red Centre, but in reality, it is the middle of the Australian Desert. I've swapped my work life with rich and famous clients to working with the indigenous first nation women of Australia. I wear shorts, sunglasses, and tramping boots. My pointed flats are in the back of my wardrobe. If I'm outside, I put a net over my head to keep the desert flies from invading my orifices, and air conditioning is essential in order to sleep at night. I'm considering buying a swag.

What is happening to me?

Little did I know that I was to meet more interesting people and have memorable experiences.

17 SIMPSONS GAP, MINI TRIPS OUT OF TOWN

From Alice Springs, Simpsons Gap is an easily accessible and a positively spiritual gap, carved out of the MacDonald ranges. There is a permanent water hole that is not for swimming but creates a reflective mirror for stunning photos. It was here I first saw the colours that even now are hard to describe, the heights that bend the neck and draw the eye to the heavens. Little rock wallabies play on the sheer cliffs. It is a place where mother nature will care for you if you sit and be still. It is a place I go to be.

I wrote:

Waves of invisible wind whisper and flow twisting their volume upwards intensifying as it wraps through unimaginable heights while blue sky is lit by the dawn.

Crispy leaves blend the harmony perfectly timed, no metronome required.

Melody rising to a crackle and rustle lifting to a crescendo then hushing to silence background music.

Rocks defining geology sing red orange rust, punctuating the natural stage.

Erupted layers once violently pushed and shoved competing for space sit powerfully staunch touching the stars.

A gap gently gifting shelter to the ancestors.

It was 26 May, 2020

A less visited site Cassia Hill, 2km from Simpsons Gap, is mostly bypassed. There is a circular walking trail which at the top takes one to Schist rock, which is 1600 million years old and is one of the oldest rock formations in Australia. Those numbers stagger me. It was here one day, as I sat alone, taking in the views, that I was visited by an ancestor. I saw him in the bush, his face clear and soft. And that was all. Nothing else happened. No words. No flashes of lightning nor windy whirls, just his presence. I sat in his presence. Then he wasn't there, but I didn't feel as though he had left.

I sang a waiata song in Te Reo Maori about love and peace.

Te aroha

Te whakapono

Me te rangimarie

Tatou tatou e

I think he was just checking me out and I was left feeling very grounded.

I thanked the ancestors, and always do when I walk their lands, then left. It was then I knew I wanted to visit Uluru. I've no idea of the connection. It was just a feeling.

It was later that week I met Ingrid.

Ingrid is a neonatal nurse, and I would often be there to see babies and mums to help with their feeding.

Ingrid is a granny hippy. A fellow Kiwi, she loves witches and fairies, all sorts of nick knacks, and although she arrived in Alice Springs with one suitcase, she had already sent two more boxes home full to the brim with "things." Her room, identical to mine but in a different building and on the top floor, was a haven for calm and peace infused with incense and aromatherapy. She had plants flowering, dreamcatchers dangling, and tie-dyed fabrics as an overlay on her tables and furniture.

As Kiwis, we connected when Ingrid was working as a neonatal nurse in the unit adjoined to Midwifery, and over a nappy change (one of the babies, not ours). We realised that we both had a few days off at the same time, and the seeds of a tiki tour (short trip) were sown. Before the week's end, we had booked a campervan and spots in Kings Canyon and Uluru National Park.

I was going to visit Uluru.

Neither of us had ever driven a camper van, but I was more than ready to give it a whirl.

The instructions for driving were emailed along with our pick-up instructions.

Reading the dimension specifications meant little to me, 7 metres long and 2.8 metres high.

Click. Download. Open.

I waited patiently for the rainbow pie wheel to stop swirling and started to read.

I was so excited, but I had a bit of anxiety building since I had gone past the motorhome yard, and eyed up what we had hired. It seemed a hell of a lot bigger than I imagined. I gulped and hid my anxiety.

The opening line in the information chapter was music to my ears

Welcome to Maui motorhomes. If this is your first time driving a camper vehicle, sit back and relax. It is very similar to driving a normal vehicle.

I wonder if it is the same as riding a bike.

Tomorrow I'll find out.

What a trip we had. This was my first holiday or journey with a new friend. We seldom had gaps in conversation, soaking in the vista while sharing stories of our lives, jobs, dreams and nightmares. We started as strangers and became friends.

The flat top of the Kings Canyon was our outlook from where we set up our campsite, pulled out the chairs and table, and popped the cork off the Oyster Bay rose. Ingrid was a dapper barbecue queen as she pulled out the plate and sizzled our sausages. In true Ingrid style, she wore her faux fur trimmed coat over her boutique top and sandals.

As the sun set, we decreed there was no place we would rather be than tucking into a beef snarler, covered in Wattie's tomato sauce, sipping bubbles from Aotearoa under the mighty skies of the Wataraka National park.

We had both left work behind, for now.

The next morning, we were up early and cranked up my Priscilla, Queen of the Desert playlist. If you have seen the film, you will know the incongruous scene of three men dressed in drag making the ascent to a lookout over Kings Canyon. This was where we were heading, a short drive to the car park and the beginning of the Rim Walk.

Nimble legged Ingrid confessed she was knackered at the top of the 500 or so steep steps that were the kill-or-cure introduction to the rest of the hike. I just nodded and smiled, unable to talk until I caught my breath! I noticed an AED (an automated external defibrillator). I didn't quite need it but was not surprised that it might come in handy.

From then on, it was a majestic climb. The trail is a six kilometre circuit passing Priscilla's Crack (yes, that is what it is called) to the first lookout across the canyon where the Drag Queens were filmed. There are sandstone domes known as The Lost City because their quirky formations give the impression of having been a town. We descended into an oasis of green called The Garden of Eden, and across the gap on a newly built bridge, then circled around to get the total view of the canyon and beyond.

Early days of coronavirus meant that Ingrid and I had the whole walk to ourselves except for a very large kangaroo who seemed to stop mid-bound on the path when he noticed us. He landed, stared at me for an indeterminable time, and bobbed off, disappearing into the rocks. He was the biggest kangaroo I had seen and the closest I had been to one in the wild, but he was gone before I had time to register fear.

Near the end of the walk, we had a conversation with an indigenous ranger who was originally from Kakadu in the north country. As part of his job, he guided the walkers along the track and checked the Automated External Defibrillator (AED) and first aid boxes, which were often used by the walkers. I mentioned to him that I may have needed the defibrillator earlier, and he confirmed that it had been used on a few occasions. I was not surprised.

The day ended with another spectacular show of natural colours as the sunset preceded a night sky full of stars and the crescent of a moon.

Ingrid had been to Uluru back when climbing it was a thing. She had been on a whistle-stop overnighter from Alice Springs with a group of young people and a lot of alcohol. Ingrid let me have my moment when I first caught sight of the amazing and iconic land mass jutting out of the flat Australian Red Centre. Words will never describe its majestic pull. I was captivated and held hostage to its red and rusty energy, not in a tangible sense, but more a visual awe. I looked towards the coloured rock as though it were an anchor.

I felt safe as I recalled the visit the ancestor had paid me back at Casia Hill. Walking the perimeter takes visitors away from some of the sacred sites and allows us to go closer to others. There were sites for women's business that had centuries-old art telling their stories, sites for men's business, and sacred sites we could not see as the path would divert away. Until being this close to Uluru, I had assumed it to be a gathering point for men's business only, its dominance portraying the masculine. It was a contemplative walk interrupted at times by groups on their Segway scooters who had tour guides sharing interesting knowledge. Ingrid and I walked independently, each with our own thoughts as company. I saw where her former climb took place. It was incredibly steep. I had no desire to climb this rock. I just needed to keep looking at it.

Beyond Uluru is Kata Tjuta, also known as The Olgas, where we went for lunch. It is like visiting the cousins of Uluru, the ones with the rowdy kids and the messy home. It sits much lower and dishevelled with an enticing array of valleys and walks. We met many walkers here, as there are varying grades from a few hundred metres to steep climbs with lookouts, sunrise viewing platforms, and sunset parks. The sacredness of this site is ever present. The dreamtime stories are mostly not disclosed to women. It was an easy place to wander through and as the sun moved across the sky, Kata Tjuta's colours transformed changing the vibrancy and shades, as though breathing life into the core.

We made our way back to our campsite then joined a tourist group for the evening. So much beauty and topped off with a very expensive dinner under the stars where we sipped Australian bubbles and ate wild game as didgeridoo tones reverberated in the background. As the sun set, it was a perfect way to recharge the nursing and midwife batteries.

Alice Springs is one of the toughest places to be a midwife. There is a government project called Closing the Gap, which aims to have less differential in health outcomes for the indigenous populations of Australia. In Alice, the gap seemed to be at its widest. The town has gentrified shops, and the streets are speckled by inequity. Frighteningly, the alcohol-infused young and old tripped and hollered their way down the paths to the grassed areas where they would eat their chicken and drink their rationed grog. At night, the kids had started the habit of throwing rocks from a sacred site, a high point overlooking an intersection where cars had to stop at the lights. The pretty funky arty town had a dark, ominous side, and nowhere else was the gap so blatantly wide. Our colleagues who worked in ED had the worst of it. There they would be subjected to abuse and filth day in and day out. Midwifery and the neonatal unit seemed to be shielded from this, but occasionally it seeped through.

Both Ingrid and I tried to keep our work lives back in Alice but eventually, as we always do, we started to debrief. We had a common patient who had touched us both...

18 EKALA

Ekala was pregnant with her second baby. She was a frail, undernourished, indigenous mum from one of the many communities. When I first met her, I was shocked at how emaciated she was. She had a history of rheumatic heart disease and gestational diabetes, and her baby on board was small. She hadn't known she was pregnant until her third trimester and didn't want to keep the baby.

Ekala's first child was in the care of family members. Alcohol was her primary nutrition, yet she was the gentlest, happiest woman. We would chat about a lot of things. Her cousin was going to help her with this baby.

The beautiful wee boy was born in a rush one evening when Ingrid was working, and she met him and cared for him until he was transferred to Adelaide via Royal Flying Doctors Service for ongoing care. He was in poor condition and returned to Alice Springs with a life-limiting prognosis. He had brain damage, most probably from his antenatal time.

He looked perfectly healthy, and his beautiful almond-shaped brown eyes were bright and would melt your heart.

Ekala had gone to Adelaide and had bonded with her son

although her cousin was his primary carer upon his return to Alice Springs. Ekala remained frail and she along with her cousin would spend many hours at his cot, until he was well enough to be discharged. The little boy was doing surprisingly well, against the odds.

Sometime later, I met them in the town centre. Ekala was pushing the pram, and her cousin was shopping. Ekala looked well. She beamed her most beautiful smile when she saw I recognised her and the baby. Her baby boy was beautiful, well-dressed, and settled in his pram.

This was more than the ordinary love that a mother had for her child. It was love against the odds.

After I left Alice Springs I learned that Ekala had died.

I've been a midwife for almost twenty years and have not been involved in maternal death. Although this is not a maternal or perinatal death, it was very sad to learn of her passing because she was a young pregnant mother I had gotten to know well.

I felt the hefty weight that is the futility of their lives.

I know her son was loved by both her and her cousin. I don't think he will be long for this life either. I still think of them. And so does Ingrid.

19 SITUATIONAL FRIENDSHIPS

I was introduced to Amy by Melissa.

Melissa was a new graduate midwife in her fifties; an Australian citizen, and originally from Korea. Melissa and I worked a couple of shifts together during my first week. She was quiet, and speaking English was challenging for her. I soon learned that Melissa was not popular at work and was the victim of classic horizontal bullying. This included colleagues judging her quality of care and mentioning it at handover, not rostering her to work in the delivery suite (DS) even though she was a new graduate and would have needed this experience, engaging in telling stories about her, and selective rostering. Rumours ran ("so I was aware") that she was a lovely person, but the aboriginals don't like her. She was slow, she wrote too much, she only came into midwifery because her friend was studying nursing and she wanted to be different: midwifery was close but different. She had poor English. She failed her midwifery and Alice Springs "gave her a chance", so she was lucky. Alice Springs were not going to keep her on. She was unsafe. It was quite a reputation.

What I came to know about Melissa was that she was also kind soul who described herself as a sheep in wolf's clothing. Melissa was married, her husband was from Mainland China, and while she chose to make Australia her home and had obtained her citizenship, he had not; but they functioned as a family. She had a grown daughter who lived in Adelaide and was studying Molecular Biology. Melissa was a housewife before starting midwifery. She chose this career because she worked as a volunteer with Refugees in Asia and was so concerned for the pregnant women, she wanted to return to these developing countries as a midwife with this skill.

Melissa said her spoken English was the hardest part of midwifery for her, as Australians were very impatient with her. She was the top academic student in her year at university. Melissa was unaware of any bullying in Alice Springs; she just thought no one liked her, and she didn't understand what bullying was. She cried when I shared with her what horizontal bullying might look like.

"That's what is happening to me," she said. "What can I do?"

Vote with your feet, was all I could recommend. At the end of her post graduate year, she did leave and found work in a busy metropolitan hospital.

Melissa lived in the staff accommodation in the other block and introduced me to Amy, a Kiwi nurse who worked in mental health.

Amy then introduced me to Tanya, another Kiwi who was also in mental health.

Amy, a stroppy and independent woman, was from the South Island, but as she quickly added, was really Australian, having moved to Sydney at the age of fourteen. She had one daughter who was estranged from her.

Surprisingly for me, (she) Amy was the first Kiwi I've met who hated New Zealand. She still owned property in Auckland where she had moved with her husband and where her daughter then lived, but was loath to return there because "it's so shit" she declared, adding to her anti Kiwi rhetoric

Amy also "can't stand Jacinda," the popular NZ exPrime Minister and her very vociferous opinion stemmed from the days Jacinda refused to give a pay rise to nurses,

I consider myself to be a fairly open person and was happy to wait and see how this friendship evolved. Amy had suggested that we go for a tiki tour on the weekend. Melissa was also invited as was another work colleague, Tanya.

I quite liked Tanya. She was a tall and attractive woman with a nice smile and she was a fellow Kiwi. We set off for what was my first tiki tour beyond the MacDonald ranges.

Tanya had an interesting story and was open and classic Kiwi. She had four children all born at home. Her former husband, a helicopter pilot, had an affair with the midwife. I was stunned and horrified but I actually found myself working up a morbid curiosity for more detail.

Our tiki tour had taken us to Rainbow valley, about an hour's drive south of Alice Springs and then a left turn onto the red dirt. It was early morning and we clambered out of the car to take photos. Melissa had never seen a dirt road.

We are so accustomed to tar seal or gravel, the sandy red road that carved its way across the desert was a picture of incredulity. Like a snow plough on a field, there is clear direction; its edges were lined with undisturbed shrubs and trees with the leaf fall and the ground cover was a sandy colour. In the distance, there were tyre tracks predominantly in the middle. Traffic was light on these roads and so most people drove left to centre. This made allowances for tyre tread and surprise encounters with wildlife, whose homes we were interrupting.

At the end of the sand track was a yellow road sign with a cross indicating a crossroad. To the right was a camping spot for freedom campers and to the left was the valley. I had seen photographic images of the rock formation announcing itself, and the reality impressed me. In this mid-morning light, it was brick red with shadowy darkness – an outcrop at one end of a vast flat valley so dry that the patchwork sands had dried and as the water was sucked into the ground underneath it, it left what looked like skin cells under the microscope.

The deep blue sky had swirls of clouds swishing high above. From where the road ended the energy of the rocks clearly beckoned us forward.

Of course, it was an aboriginal gathering spot. This site was mainly occupied and used for ceremonies when the rains came. In the wet season, seeds were gathered and crushed in grindstones to make bread. Stone tools were used for scraping and cutting. When it dried up, the indigenous would move on to find permanent waterholes elsewhere.

We were free to wander into the rocky area in certain parts with signage directing us to keep clear of areas of special interest or sacred sites. In front of the outcrop was a vast flat deserted circular expanse. How wonderful it would be to see the water flowing through here.

It was as we were walking around this space that Tanya engaged Melissa and I with her story. Clearly, I was intrigued, but sadly really, as I found it all very uncomfortable being a midwife and imagining that this midwife had crossed a professional boundary.

But I became curiouser and curiouser. Tanya spoke about how her trusted midwife for two of her three births, began an emotional affair with the husband. This further developed with time, and they eventually ended up together. Melissa was listening intently and when she and I were walking side by side, she asked if it was ok that I had been asking so many questions. Perhaps I had been overcurious but as it turned out Tanya had clearly told the story before and provided an entertaining insight.

"What is an emotional affair?" Melissa asked. Thinking back to our talk about horizontal bullying I was not as surprised to learn she didn't know what this might mean. Cultural nuances were evident. We were back in the vehicle at this stage. Amy, Tanya and I all gave our slant on emotional affairs. I kept it simple and said a relationship that has everything but the sex. Amy added – that's so they can pretend it isn't happening.

Melissa looked shocked and later confided in me that she didn't think that happened in her home country.

As we left Rainbow valley, the light had changed colours, so the rock formation looked as though it had been turned to face the sun.

As we were on a Tiki tour, we were all keen to discover more, so instead of heading home to the austerity of the nursing home, we turned west onto the Ernest Giles Road to view the Henbury Meteorite Reserve. This road was more gravelly than red sand, yet as isolated as the one to Rainbow valley. There were no other travellers.

Henbury Meteorites Conservation Reserve contains twelve craters which were formed when a meteor hit the earth's surface 4,700 years ago. The Henbury Meteor, weighing several tonnes and accelerating to over 40,000 km per hour, disintegrated before impact, and the fragments formed the twelve craters

The information sign said *tjintu waru tjinka yapu tjinka kurdaitcha kuka*, which roughly translates in the Luritja language as 'a fiery devil ran down from the Sun and made his home in the Earth. He will burn and eat any bad blackfellows.' This indicates a living memory of the event.

It is a crossroad for many language groups, although the indigenous would not ever camp close by. It is considered a sacred site to the Arrernte people and would have formed during human habitation of the area.

Australia is full of such scientifically significant information and attracts geologists and astronautical experts from all around the world.

Of note was Eugene Shoemaker who had co-discovered the Comet Shoemaker-Levy 9 that crashed into Jupiter causing a massive "scar" on the face of the planet.

Eugene Shoemaker was studying these impact craters and died on the Tanami Track just up the road from Alice Springs in 1997.

The fatal crash happened when Hale-Bopp was still visible to the naked eye, had passed perihelion and moved into the southern celestial hemisphere.

Some of his ashes were carried to the moon. Shoemaker is the only person whose remains have been placed on any celestial body outside Earth

I think of him when I look at the night sky.

RIP Eugene Shoemaker.

20 KINGS CANYON CAMPING

Living in the nurse's hostel was a flashback to my student nursing days of the 80s. When a fellow Kiwi nurse asked me to go camping to celebrate her birthday, it was an opportunity not to be missed.

Tanya had been on the Rainbow valley trip, and we had gotten along well. Having been intrigued by her story, I was also fascinated by how she could have left her sons home with her parents.

It's the way of the outback world that for every person you meet, (if they are not locals), they have a story to match their personality.

Tanya had been a mature student in New Zealand and was seven years post qualification. With a tall and sturdy build, she had a booming personality to match. To me she looked rather out of place in her denim jeans, leather belt, and matching boots with a black Akubra hat to finish the uniform.

I say uniform as it was what all the mental health nurses wore. A Kiwi seeing a Kiwi looking like a cattle musterer off a station, was odd.

With the look and an attitude to match, Tanya seemed to have men at her fingertips. It was her birthday, and she had invited me to join a large crew on a camping weekend. It sounded like a hoot.

There were going to be four carloads, colleagues of the birthday girl and people she had networked with during her first three weeks in the "Springs" which is how she referred to Alice Springs. Her birthday was on a Monday, so she suggested we all take a day's leave. Kings Canyon was chosen as the venue. It was a five hour drive from Alice Springs.

Tanya came to me after work one day and asked me not to mention the trip to Melissa. She found her too difficult to talk to. Not on the same page. I was surprised at her frankness, but it was her birthday after all.

The week before we travelled, I was checking about what we were to bring and making plans for the walks. Tanya was a little on edge, but said, "Oh, we are not planning too much, it will all be ok, just bring whatever."

Kiwis are often very fluid with plans, but I sensed a flippancy that was more exclusive than inclusive, so I said, "If your plans have changed, just let me know - I don't have to go."

She dismissed this, but followed by asking, "Are you ok to travel with Amy?"

Without waiting for me to answer, she tumbled into a tirade, warning me to be wary of Amy. She cautioned me about her moods and implied that her non drinking "had a history."

She was inferring she wasn't just a non-drinker – but probably had a problem with it. I was filled in with how disruptive Amy was in the office and how she thought she was much better than everyone else. "Oh, she's ok," said Tanya, "just be wary of her."

"A few of the others aren't coming because of her," she continued. "They don't want to come because she's so moody and negative. And she is very 'judgy' about smoking and drinking."

"Are you sure you want me to go?" I asked Tanya. "Oh yeah, it's all good. No worries. Just don't let on that you know."

Know what? I wondered. What did Tanya think of Amy?

I assured her that I would not say anything to Amy.

It might be an interesting trip.

Driving any distance in the outback is best done very early in the morning. I told Amy that I would be set to go by six. She wouldn't be ready before nine she replied.

I was the passenger, so I just needed to go with the flow. We packed the vehicle, but the camping gear needed to be secured, and the new ropes did not fit the Rav 4 she owned. After getting new straps and a coffee, we finally left Alice Springs at about 11am.

The others left after one of the blokes finished work at 2pm. So much for us all taking annual leave, I thought. We were supposed to have gotten there early to find a good camping spot.

The doubts that this trip would not be fun soon disappeared when we were on our way. As a passenger, this time I saw the landscape with more detail and was fascinated again by the wonderful vista.

I was looking forward to setting up my swag and tent and re-exploring the Canyon.

The conversation with Amy was easy, but she started to share her opinion of Tanya not long into the journey. No holds barred; she let rip with tales from work, citing control issues, self-opinionated arrogance, and ignorance.

Colleagues who had been invited, had confided that they had changed their minds and were not coming because Tanya and the lads would be drinking and smoking all weekend.

Two delightfully different versions. I said nothing. Just nodded and agreed.

I started to wish I hadn't come.

By way of distraction, I asked Amy if she wanted to be adventurous and go the dirt road, which was fewer kilometres, but would take about the same time.

I hadn't anticipated her reluctance to travel over 20kmph on the flat dirt road. However, we eventually got to the Canyon and had the delights of seeing a caravan of camels on the way.

The campground had plenty of van spots, but less suitable tent sites. There were fire pits in random places, and we orientated ourselves so we could be close to amenities and have a view across to the Canyon. Most of the ablutions and kitchens were closed. This was the coronavirus response to falling tourist numbers and low staffing. We found the best camping spot where we could all have space but share the fire pit. We had a magical view of the place we would walk the next day.

Tanya and the others arrived shortly after we set up our camp. Their numbers had reduced to five, so they travelled together. Tanya said hello but scoured the campsite, looking for a better spot. I was so annoyed and yet I had mentally predicted that she would not want to have had a camp spot chosen for her. Jeremy, who was driving, came over. I was very polite yet firm when I said, "How bizarre that Tanya feels the need to camp on the other side of the grounds. It's quite offensive, to be honest."

They came back and set up, as far as politely possible from Amy.

This was the beginning of what turned out to be a passive-aggressive few days. I was stuck in the middle of two colleagues pretending to like each other but obviously, they did not. I felt like a mute referee as each confided in anecdotes about the other.

I was becoming quite good at non-engagement and found it amusing.

My escape plan was to keep myself busy with walks, reading, and sipping Prosecco. In such a grand environment, it's easy to do.

I became an observer of human behaviour. I know midwives have a reputation for being a forceful gaggle when together, but five mental health nurses were mind-blowing. Each was clamouring over the other with anecdotes of situations, clients, and colleagues, all with the undertones of ego-centric notions of how they were such amazing support for their clients. Jargon was thrown about like a netball.

The controlling personality of Tanya was intriguing. I sensed some sexual tension between Jeremy, who had quit his third marriage, moved interstate and would do whatever Tanya suggested, and Mick, an Irishman, who undisputedly liked the 'demon drink.'

Amy had already shared the gossip that Tanya had slept with another colleague; so I was curious to see what the state of the nation was with two of the camping team. She was a flirt, after all. The other more senior nurse was Rawiri, a Maori, slightly older than the others, who seemed to be a quiet observer and had little to say. He was married and seemed confidently reserved, though he could certainly stack away the liquor without becoming a larrikin.

We pooled our tables and food and set up around a fire pit under the broad sweep of clear blue skies. We meandered to the lookout within the camping grounds and watched the sun setting over the mighty King's Canyon, grateful for the coronavirus keeping the crowds of visitors away. Dusk heralded the milky way.

There was a subtle simmering tension within the gathering, the odd contradiction and accentuated speech. I was really hoping there would be no blow up of these formidable personalities.

But we shared an easy meal and, after an early night, were up at pre-dawn the next day. There are rules about when you can walk these walks, and we had to be off the canyon rim by 11am so that the heat would not kill us. I had warned them about how steep the ascending steps were and reassured them that there was a defibrillator and emergency equipment waiting at the top of the climb.

I don't think they believed me.

We had a fantastic day. There was enough civility for us all to enjoy the Kings Canyon walk, and no one was pushed over the edge physically or metaphorically.

That evening, back around the fire, we were talking and laughing. I thought that all was not as bad as I had imagined. We seemed to be having a great time; being with nature is always a blessing. Tongues loosened and voices were raised. Amy shushed the voices a couple of times but they ignored her and finally Amy found it all too much and took herself off to the isolation of the tent.

Tanya seemed irritated at this independent behaviour and became verbally abusive in her absence.

I chose to pretend to be oblivious to the disharmony. It warranted a little bit of selective hearing I thought.

Then our group breached the etiquette of Kings Canyon Camping ground. The laughter and noise upset the family near us - we had all watched them erect their double swag for the parents and two singles for the pre school-age kids. Daddy bear came over to ask us to be quiet; after all, it was past 9pm.

The booming male voices and female cackles were quiet for some time, and I took my leave and snuggled into my tent.

The quiet didn't last long as the smoking and whiskey swirling continued. There are no secrets in a camping ground. Even if the conversations were muted, they were clearly audible, and I, too, was aware of the disruption into the wee hours. The little group of mental health nurses was letting their hair down after a stressful week. Apparently, it was their right. Apparently.

Tension was palpable the next morning when Amy joined us for breakfast.

The lads were preparing a cook-up. Their hangovers needed to soak up the food. Amy mentioned papa bear's visit and defended the family while accusing the lads with bleary eyes of being far too loud. This set off a cascade of disquiet as each supported their opinion.

That was about all Tanya could cope with. She had the annoying habit of always having a text conversation on the go while talking with the group. With an obvious hangover, her black dyed hair hung like a witch's wig, and she cracked first. Over a bacon buttie, she announced they, being her carload, would go home a day early. Suddenly needing to phone her children in New Zealand, and friends wanting to meet for dinner and, and, and...

'The lady doth protest too much,' was my thought.

I was initially disappointed, but after the next scenario that unfolded, I was relieved.

Another verbal scuffle about the night before started.

Amy was so annoyed at the sudden change of plans and what she perceived to be inappropriate behaviour the night before, that she started clearing up the breakfast and packing away her table and equipment. She scraped what appeared to be the leftovers into the fire pit and went to wash up.

The lads were still eating breakfast.

I watched in disbelief as a grown man pulled a long rasher of bacon from the ashes of the fire and stuffed it into his mouth to prove to Amy that they hadn't finished eating. The Irishman sucked the ash-covered bacon rind, and grease dripped onto his 'Guinness is Great' t-shirt. Then, with theatrical effect, wiped his mouth with the back of his hand and said, "Now I'm finished."

This was better than any sitcom I had watched in a while. I took my time with my cuppa as an awkward silence descended.

I spotted Rawiri heading over to the lookout, so I joined him.

"Might be a long trip home for both of us," I said. He nodded and said nothing. We let enough time pass so the dust would have settled back at camp.

I got my book out and settled in for some reading as Tanya's team packed up with timely efficiency. We all said our goodbyes as if we were the best of friends.

I couldn't help but say, "Think of us when you are tucking into your Heineman's dinner, we're having sausages again." The boys didn't make eye contact. Tanya just grinned a stupid grin, and Rawiri drove off.

I told Amy that they were meeting their other colleagues who didn't want to come camping at the restaurant for a birthday meal.

Amy was seething but said in a cool voice, "I don't give a damn," and I don't think she did.

Kings Canyon, in the middle of Australia, was delightful to visit and walk through. Sunrise and sunset evolved and captivated each time. This canyon radiated sacredness. The ash-coated bacon butty demonstration will take a long time to forget. If I ever need to seek professional help from mental health nurses, I'll just take a moment to remember, and I'm sure I will feel immediately better.

Tanya's and my path would cross again, and the next time wouldn't be quite as harmonious.

As for a camping trip with a group of mental health nurses, well, it did seem a good idea at the time.

21 THE PRISONER...THINGS YOU SEE THAT YOU WISH YOU HADN'T.

My accommodation was onsite, so rarely did I bother going to the canteen. Coronavirus had ensured a one-way food purchase system and plenty of seats with tables outside to sit for our break. I needed a coffee and Mimi, who was a good barista, had returned from leave. I ordered my coffee and sat outside under the coloured sail-like cloth, sun protectors strung across the courtyard in a bright and happy way. The fresh air was easy to breathe, and the blue sky always left me feeling grateful for a good climate.

My sense of gratitude and peace were shattered by the parading of a prisoner through the courtyard into the radiology department.

It seemed like a long journey for this man; he had both his hands cuffed at his front. He wore a desert-coloured jumpsuit that had the fabric tucked in such a way that his lower leg was protected; the shackle was on the outside.

He was indigenous. I could see blood across his ear, dried and matted into a thick mess accentuated by his slouched posture, hung head, and shuffling steps.

It was pitiful.

Beside him, was the woman prison officer with her blue gloved hand, held firmly to his elbow, her colleague taller and younger than she, gripped the prisoner's forearm in what seemed to be a tight hold, and both led him to the back entrance of Radiology.

The shackles and the shuffling haunted me. Surely this old and feeble man could pose no threat to the public. Surely handcuffs would suffice.

I had accepted the reality of a temporary lifestyle change, but had sure knowledge that I would soon be going back to London. I intended to make the most of my time in the desert.

During my first week in the hostel accommodation, I was two doors along from a nurse who had a beautiful sign on her door saying she was on night duty - a reminder for others to be quiet during the day. When I first met her, we were in the kitchen and we exchanged simple pleasantries and basic introductions. The standard information sharing invariably includes what department, how long have you been there and when are you leaving. Nothing else matters and so many people cross our paths in these communities it is of little interest to invest in a friendship. I thought Maria was a nice person, she was a regular to Alice. Her physical features and mannerisms reminded me of my friend in Highgate. We started to bump into each other frequently and a friendship began.

Maria's dad was Greek, so she is Greek. To her horror, I confessed that I had thought of her as Jewish, and it has now become our delightful joke that she is my Jewish friend.

Maria felt she was from a Kibbutz in a former life. I said she must have been in the desert too long.

We spent many an hour debriefing from our respective shifts, laughing and gossiping, which was all part of being grounded and staying relatively sane in a challenging environment.

Her friendship has lasted beyond the walls of the hospital accommodation and we have vowed to meet in the Mediterranean on one of her family's islands, drink ouzo while we solve the problems of the world.

I wrote this limerick for her.

Maria
There once was a Nurse based in Alice
Whose dorm room was decked like a palace
But next to the loo
She could hear all the poo
Going down the old pipe-like chalice.

22 KARLU KARLU - GETTING AWAY FROM IT ALL

No matter where you live, there is always that commonality where you get up, go to work, come home, go to sleep, and repeat. Some days it dawns with more punch where you are. I had that moment after being in Alice Springs for about a month. I had been caught up in the newness of the town, the short and memorable trips about the region, and although every day it was warm with golden hues of colour, I had a moment where I woke up to the slap of reality.

I couldn't hop on the Eurostar but could drive somewhere alone and have some space. That irony was not lost in my thoughts.

I booked into the Devil's Marbles hotel for two nights on a budget donga. It is a four hour drive north, and close to an indigenous site called Karlu Karlu. Of course, I'd be keen to visit it. I could eat at the hotel; I could write, sleep, and read...

I'm not sure what was going on in my head and heart as I packed my bag. I opened my Paris styled carry aboard that has been on all my European trips. Firstly, I put on my shorts but changed into my travel clothes, dusted off the chic city shoes and packed a pair of sandals, some earrings and wearable art, a Samuel Coraux necklace, lipstick and my Prada sunglasses. The devil wears Prada even at the Marbles. Maybe it's a sign. More of a sigh, I felt.

I felt that my proverbially clipped wings had grown feathers as I headed north for the first time. Not far out of Alice, I saw the Tanami Road leading to Halls Creek. This surprised me, and I had yet another moment to readjust my reality radar - I had been to Halls Creek back in 2007; my brother had lived there for almost twenty years, but I hadn't factored that this road connected the wild and remote Kimberly district to the Central desert. I took a photo of the sign to send to my brother when I got some mobile reception.

I thought that I was as far away from London as I could ever get. It was probably correct.

My first stop was Barrow Creek, where Peter Falconio met his fate (apparently). Or did his girlfriend, who was 'communicating' with another bloke, actually get rid of him? An ABC television programme earlier in the week had just revisited this case of the British backpacker murdered in the outback twenty years ago. The twenty eight year old was shot dead when he and his girlfriend Joanne Lees were ambushed near Barrow Creek in 2001. His body was never found. Alice Springs has plenty of theories about this event.

My recollection of the event followed a trip with my brother to Wolfe Creek Crater in Western Australia years ago. Wolfe Creek is a fascinating place of natural interest as one of the biggest meteorite crater sites in the world. BB told me there was a Wolfe Creek film I should watch.

I bought the DVD and sat with my kids, who were too young to watch it. It was an engrossing, terrifying, yet captivating film that still fills me with terror. Now all these years later, I had the same rush of adrenalin as I came to Barrow Creek, and I was less than easy when I was followed by a white utility vehicle just as I left the town.

The same scenario as the murder mystery. Seriously, I couldn't make that up! Of course, white utility vehicles are a dime a dozen here in the desert, and the farmer soon overtook me and was gone. I did keep checking my rear view mirror, though.

Then, because driving in the desert at 130 kpm could seem boring, the next town claimed to be the UFO capital of Australia.

UFO sightings have been part of Wycliffe Well's folklore since World War II, and the town's reputation for the unexplained attracts all types, even the Royal Australian Air Force has stopped in to investigate.

Two model aliens sit in front of the Wycliffe Well Holiday Park to welcome travellers. The Park's owner says that many claim to have seen UFOs zipping around the night sky. The pub has reputedly the biggest range of beer available in Australia. Maybe this is a contributing factor in the UFO sightings.

I did manage to poke my face into an ET-type frame and do a selfie. I couldn't bring myself to have an alien cup of tea in the tearoom.

The Devils Marbles Hotel has a row of rusted old cars and tractors lining the entrance, along with the palm trees that simulate an oasis. It is an oasis of sorts and as I made my way to my donga, I passed an impressive inside restaurant and an outside area with wooden tables and chairs invitingly situated around the pool.

I had booked a single room, and not for the first time realised that this is a rookie mistake as the toilet and shower block, although very clean, is in a donga next door.

I went back and doubled the cost but booked a chalet. It also had a tv which I watched as there was no Wi-Fi or phone connection. I felt rather guilty that I couldn't cope without modern technology for two days.

I settled into the room and had a swim.

I dressed for dinner. Simply of course as I didn't have any flash clothes anyway, but I did wear my sling back pointy toe shoes.

The mozzies[1] found me outside in the balmy evening as the sun set. Carloads of indigenous locals arrived at the hotel bar, and many were turned away. They know how it is. If they have caused trouble with the grog, they are not allowed in. The bartender, who is a Canadian living with a cattle owner (lucky her), skilfully noted the sober drivers and rationed them to one drink. They kept trying to buy more grog². She called over one of the women who sorted it out. That's the way here. There are rules, and there are rule breakers.

Sadly, the results of alcohol with the indigenous does not end well.

For a while, country music played in the background. The triple award-winning restaurant was filled with people from God knows where and randomly, I had 3G on my phone that came and went. I had a sneaky feeling that I might have arrived here by accident, but the desert was growing on me.

Dawn slipped into daylight unimpeded by clouds so the day arrived speedily. I set out early to visit Karlu Karlu and continued on to Tennant creek for a nosey.

As you rejoin the Stuart Highway and get further from the hotel, you will come across a valley with thousands of red-brown granite boulders of various sizes, some as big as six metres across. These boulders are over 150 million years old and are imposing and fascinating to look at. Some of them are split cleanly while others are small, round, and playful. Some of the larger ones seem to defy gravity and challenge physics as they sit precariously on top of one another. How is this even possible?

This area is also significant in terms of dream time stories. One of the most popular stories involves the ancestor Arrange, who once walked through the area and left behind a maid hair-string belt, a traditional garment worn by initiated Aboriginal men.

I walked gently and purposefully along the paths that weaved in and out of the rocks. In some places the elders ask that you do not take photos, other places that you do not climb. Karlu Karlu has a calming effect on your soul.

A family arrived, two young children with their parents. We got chatting and sharing our story of how we were in Karlu Karlu during the pandemic. They had sold their house and bought a boat and were now confined even on the seas to where they could travel. The dad in his early 40's said to me, "We spend less so we don't have to work so hard". A gem of wisdom shared at the marbles.

As if an alarm sounded, the flies arrived. Within a short few minutes, I was cloaked in small annoying mites that cling to your skin, climb into your ears and up your nose. Eating them is always by accident. I wrapped my rainbow-coloured silk chiffon scarf I had bought from Grazyna's boutique in Highgate village, covering my head and face, winning the battle for now. I would return at dusk. It is not a place you can just call past. It is a sacred place that needs to be experienced.

Tennant Creek was just one hour north of Karlu Karlu. The town had a reputation that was not inviting, but many of our pregnant women came to Alice Springs to birth, so it was good for me to know where their home was. My first impressions were a pleasant surprise. There is a main street and what looked like a cultural centre, couple of pubs and a café. I bought a wine glass in Vinny's charity shop and had a delicious coffee before returning to the sanctuary of my retreat at the oasis in the desert.

I didn't let it happen too often but when it hit, it hit bad. Pining for my former life.

Through rose-tinted glasses, I would sit and look at my photos with my London friends, my trips to Italy or Belgium, and my mates in Ireland. I would be overwhelmed with grief and loss and a sense of homesickness that I knew had no cure. It used to happen to me when I first moved to Ireland; then I pined for Aotearoa, New Zealand, my house, my job, my my my, me me me... My adult children were the best at making me accountable for my own happiness.

Difficult to fully appreciate here in the middle of Australia. But Covid was rampant in the UK. "Mum, it's shit here," Vinny would say. "Stay where you are; at least you are safe, and you can go outside." I watched the news. More and more of my London Whānau were catching coronavirus and recovering, but it hit them hard. I listened as my friend Rose told me that three of her work colleagues had died. That sobered me up.

Then, after some time, and plenty of FaceTime calls, it would pass. I knew it would revisit, but I would see the desert with fresh eyes and again count my blessings that I was in the most magical spot in the world.

23 TENANT CREEK

As my contract finished in Alice, I was offered a new placement in Tennant Creek. It was Midwifery Group Practice, Monday - Friday with on-call to cover obstetric emergencies. I packed up my nursing home room and was delighted to be heading north. When the borders with Western Australia eventually re opened and were mapped out, I would go the high road up and across via Broome then down. That thought made me feel as though I was closer to my siblings in Perth at least.

I was, on one hand, fully aware of how the pandemic was interrupting the lives of millions, all the Zoom talk was about the news in Italy and London where many friends and family were locked down and isolated. On the other hand, I was spectacularly alone in the middle of the desert.

Lucky, yes. Lonely, yes.

I made the conscious decision to engage with colleagues and the community to keep myself balanced

When I arrived in Tennant Creek, I knew it had a bad reputation for being a town with high rates of sexual abuse, and it had been in the news recently of three teenage girls burning down the supermarket. The only food source was a pop-up shed. However, the hospital where I stayed had private single rooms with patios, a well-maintained pool outside, and security gates around the compound.

Despite the town's reputation, I found the atmosphere within the hospital to be friendly and upbeat, thanks to the presence of a number of long-term staff and locals who provided stability and continuity that is often lacking in remote areas. The hospital also had the best educational centre that I had seen and if given the chance, I would go back there without hesitation.

I was invited to the Barkley Women's Sip and Paint event. I had no idea who these women were, and I knew I couldn't paint, but I sure as hell could sip.

I booked myself into the homestead accommodation and made my way after work on a Friday, full of that old familiar spirit of independence and travel.

The roadhouse was another oasis, the land well-groomed and watered, so the grass was inviting and green. There was a pool, and the motel rooms were modern and comfortable. A large bar restaurant area already had customers when I arrived. I joined them.

The women arrived by plane, by 4X4, by utility vehicle, singularly, and some with a carload.

Most went straight to the bar, then with a drink in hand, joined the large table acknowledging familiar faces, long-time friends, and newcomers.

This could have been any gathering of women in any café or restaurant in any town or city. What made this different is that the Barkly Homestead Sip and Paint event was for the women of the Barkley district, an unimaginably vast area in Australia's centre, one-third bigger than the UK. Most of the women were from the cattle stations, having driven up to eleven hours, much of it on dirt roads or by flying their own plane.

For this weekend, they would leave their families to fend for themselves, swap the saddle-worn jeans and dust for frocks and makeup, their RM Williams boots for stilettos, and indulge in good food and wine with like-minded women.

I quietly observed the arrivals, intrigued at what they wore, later learning about Pinctada pearls and pink diamonds, and listening to eye-watering values.

Whilst enjoying the fashions and artistic flare, I chatted in the meet-and-greet manner, feeling instantly comfortable and knowing I was about to have my good spirits topped up. I sipped on Australian Prosecco, contemplating how unimaginable this would have been a year ago as I travelled from Heathrow, embarking on my six-month working holiday in Australia.

All the clichés of coronavirus fit my story. I wasn't sure these women really knew or needed to know about the pandemic. Their isolation was an invisible protective barrier. I would challenge any coronavirus to survive where these women lived.

I was seated next to Sue and was engrossed in her story. Sue is a bore runner who had travelled eleven hours to be here. A bore runner is a person who drives around the station, usually two or three times a week, checking the water for cattle. The water can be in dams or natural waterholes, but it is often underground water that needs to be pumped by a windmill, solar, or diesel motor. Her's was the first of many intriguing station tales I was to hear over the weekend.

As time passed, I became distracted by the presence of a newcomer who sat opposite us, perhaps because she did not seem to fit the profile I had seen thus far.

Marg was wearing grey shorts and a polo neck shirt that was buttoned one from the top. Her grey, un-styled hair was pulled back by an Alice band. No earrings or lipstick. Her hands had rings, some with semi-precious stones, on each digit.

Lining her forehead were deep wrinkles. Her cheeks hung softly but merged into a bulbous neck that may have hidden a goitre.

She sipped her coffee, which had been sweetened by three sugar sticks and she proceeded to add another and stirred.

I was mesmerised. Now satisfied, her caffeine was to taste, her lower jaw tucked in giving the appearance she needed her dentures fitted, her right cheek pulled up into a double bulb, closing her right eye. The lower left side of her mouth gaped.

A non-binary Popeye was sitting at my table.

Snapping me from my thoughts, she was introduced around the table. Yes, we have met, she said as my name was given to her. I smiled as if I remembered but was so grateful, I hadn't swapped my sunglasses for regular because I could be incognito in my thoughts for a moment.

Showing no awareness of social cues, the newcomer spoke over the lovely Kate, who had also just joined the table. Ms Popeye needed to tell us about how her wallet had just been stolen.

Well, I had my purse stolen right out of my bag from the Memo on Thursday. She pulled out her grubby white cloth carry bag with TCWI (Tennant Creek Women's Institute) logo and presented it to the table as if it were evidence. I got it back, of course.

"With all the cash gone, I expect?" said polite Kate.

"No, she took the cash. I only had twenty bucks, but she tapped twice at the BP. She bought toilet paper and coke. She stole my wallet and just bought toilet paper! She tried to get money from Westpac. But the cops got her. She was on CCTV wasn't she? And I know her. One of the indigenous women who calls me Aunty. I'll call her Aunty. She won't be calling me Aunty when I read my victim impact statement at court on Thursday. She'll get a first-class ticket to nowhere if I have anything to say about it."

There was a silence that was awkward to fill. Popeye didn't seem to notice and slurped her coffee before excusing herself to go outside for a fag. The proverbial penny dropped. The memo! Now I knew where I had met this woman. She had been one of only four people to have dressed up for the "Logies-themed quiz night" a week previously. My buddy had dressed as Steve Irvine, and I had become Shazza, aka Sharon Strzelecki from Kath n Kim, an iconic Australian sitcom. We had nailed the fancy dress yet had been "robbed of the prize" by a she-man posing as a sound technician, the only fancy dress being headphones and clipboard.

It was much fun later sharing our tragic, unfair story over bubbles. All for a laugh, Shazza and Steve realised that the only way to win a prize at the Memo was to be a local and ugly, and neither of us planned to stay that long in Tennant Creek to achieve either status.

As more interesting, strong, and independent station women arrived at the Homestead, donned in stylish clothes radiating their intention of having a fabulous time, the Prosecco flowed. I was able to avoid Popeye for the weekend.

I learned about cattle stations and their staggeringly huge land mass. Drovers are experienced stockmen and women who move the livestock over long distances. The ringers round up the stock. Out stations, mustering and drafting.

I've learned that the women of the stations work hard and play hard.

When scrolling through their photos on their phones, there are photos of beef stock and bore holes.

Flood waters can isolate their stations for weeks at a time, and their mail is delivered weekly by plane. They have to be strong, and they have to be resilient.

The sip and paint was not just about the obvious. It was about community, connectedness, and camaraderie.

These women look after each other even though they live days apart.

My new artistic talent, as evidenced on canvas the next morning, will be packed in my bag as I leave Australia.

Sip and Paint at the Barkley homestead was a bit of magic in my sojourn in the Aussie sunshine.

24 WEIRD AND WONDERFUL PEOPLE AND PLACES

I had already figured out that rural Australian towns attracted all sorts of people. The born and bred locals are a rarity in the workforce. There are the Asian immigrants who have to work in rural settings to fulfil their visa conditions, then there were the semi-retired who are travelling around Australia on a working holiday. Many are here for the money sending sizeable amounts back to New Zealand or Ireland for mortgage deposits. Then there are those who are divorced and broke or just don't fit into city workplaces and for one reason or another probably wouldn't get a job in a metro hospital.

It is highly improbable that a midwife/ nurse or any health professional comes to the outback of Australia for altruistic motives. Money is the driver and in fairness, the isolation along with the social inequity and cultural norms of the clientele are the most challenging and people need to be financially rewarded. To a point that is. What disturbed me was that over time I have accidentally been the confidante to healthcare workers' actual motivation, and it is distressing.

One such example was Tanya, whom I had become friends with but after the Kings Canyon camping trip, I had quietly distanced myself from her and had decided to take a temporary position in

Tennant Creek. I was secretly disappointed as the five hour drive between towns would have meant the friendship would easily fade away. Before I knew it, (in fact, the same weekend as I travelled up), Tanya too had arrived and was on my doorstep excited about her new position with the mental health team. It had become vacant after the previous post holder had committed suicide and Tanya had been the only person to put her hand up to fill the position.

Every night after work, Tanya came to my hospital-provided accommodation (one of the best I had ever had), to use the pool and "partake of a debrief" as she put it, as her "team" were so difficult to worth with.

Over the first five visits she emptied my Hennessy and I regretted introducing her to my tipple. But as Kiwis go, we look out for each other and although I recognised a resentment building within me, one month would soon be over.

However, after a couple more weeks of this habit, I was weary of the visits and craved a quiet space after work. One of the boys from Alice Springs who had been on the camping trip had scheduled a visit. I was looking forward to a social catch up with him, but the bizarre behaviour of Tanya meant that I was not going to meet him at all. I was not included in the brunch or dinner plans, and upon my suggestion to meet for the Sunday morning walk, it was dismissed.

After he returned to Alice Springs, the old habit returned. One more time only. When she confided that she needed J, her friend and colleague, to vouch for her as she was going to apply for the team leader position in Tennant Creek, it all made sense. From my perspective, I felt the town and service needed someone with more mental health experience, but Tanya declared that the team were all useless and besides the pay was amazing, "I will be able to pay for the boarding fees and keep my new car".

I told her I thought she was punching above her weight. She smiled and said, "Well, it may as well be me getting that salary as anyone." A calculating mercenary and Peter Principal combo. What could go wrong?

I have long suspected the concept of Peter Principle to be endemic in the outback. The Peter Principle is an observation that the tendency in most organisational hierarchies, such as that of a corporation, is for every employee to rise in the hierarchy through promotion until they reach a level of respective incompetence. I was shocked at how overt this situation was; but it seemed to have happened.

I feared for the mental health services in Tennant Creek.

Ms Mae was one of the weird nurses I came across. She was part Māori, in her early fifties and had OCD evidenced by the manner in which she straightened the chairs in the waiting room every morning, and every lunchtime. She lived in the hospital accommodation with her teenage daughter. No one ever saw the daughter as she hid away in her room, hating living in the middle of Australia. Mae was popular with those who didn't work directly with her, but a nightmare to have to share clinical space with. The over-exuberant gush of compliments she vomited out on our first meeting made me wary, and within a few days she had passed on gossip and warnings about colleagues whom I had found to be quite sound.

But as a fellow Kiwi, who would gladly greet her with a *Kia Ora* each morning, I was invited into her fold; it was like being in the popular group at school. I was on Ms Mae's team.

On a particular Friday, I had been invited by Mae to one of the GP's flats to watch an All Blacks versus Australia Test match. It was by special invite, and *could I not mention it* to this one and that one, that Dr Dajid was going to record it and we were going to order pizza. Rav is from Pakistan and when I said to Ms Mae, I was surprised he followed rugby, she fluffed it off with a, "Oh he's got the sports channels, he won't mind."

So I was right, Dajid probably doesn't follow rugby.

As my friends and family will attest, I am a bit of a rugby nut, so I was delighted to be watching the All Blacks with fellow supporters and it felt good to be doing something social.

On the day of the game, I went into work to print off some all-black flags to fly. Mae was in her office . We met in the coffee room.

"Oh I met another Kiwi nurse and her Irish friend, who are coming this afternoon. She is lovely," said Mae looking across her shoulder at me.

"That would be Tanya and Mick ? They are mental health nurses, aye," I said rhetorically.

Mae was, I felt, a bit annoyed that I knew these two already. I then nailed the first nail into my coffin.

I said, "Yes, I know them quite well. I used to be good friends of theirs." There can be a hierarchy of ownership in these friendships/work colleagues. They become a clique in rural locations and again like school kids playgrounds, become a venue for bullying by exclusion.

An imperceptible twitch accompanied Mae's next question.

"Oh what do you mean, used to be?"

I proffered a short version

"I upset Tanya when I questioned her suitability for the role she had applied for here in TC (Tennant Creek), because she had only been registered a few years and I felt the mental health management role would need someone more experienced."

"We registered the same year," Ms Mae said with a hint of indignation.

"Oops," I thought.

I didn't get into Tanya's bizarre behaviour on our camping trip, nor the fact that her first week in the town was spent shagging an engineer whose wife was still in Alice Springs, or the reality that she needed "debriefing" every day after work, emptying my two bottles of Hennessy in one week.

Not that we had a falling out at all, but I made my point that even though she thought the department was desperate for a manager after the previous gentleman had committed suicide, I didn't think she was experienced enough and that it was slightly unethical to be in a job just for the enticing salary to pay her children's boarding school fees.

Tanya had told me that she thought they would be lucky to have her. She had heard the service was shite but she would chance it and apply. She could do it for a year (the usual rationalisation of what money could be earned) which was a rhetoric I had heard on other occasions.

I explained to Ms Mae that I thought that Tanya was punching above her weight, but hats off to her if she thought she could get away with it

"I don't want any awkwardness at rugby" said Ms Mae. I'll have to tell her you are coming. She stated.

Tongue in cheek, I replied, "let's just keep it a surprise."

I was going to enjoy this. Tanya could be good company and it would be good to meet up with Mick. So I sent a friendly text to Tanya to say that I'd be seeing her at Dajid's for the rugby, and didn't think much more of it. I was far too busy choosing an All Black flag to print off, and finding a small stick to sellotape it to.

Later that morning I got a phone call from Mae.

"I've been very upset by what you said about Tanya. Very upset and I am very uncomfortable that you are going to be there, so I have decided that I would prefer that you don't come."

It took me a moment or two to realise what she meant.

"I'm uninvited ?" I asked

"Yes, I hope you don't mind," she said.

What the fuck I thought, but I just quietly said, "Ummm OOOO KKKKK," and without actually saying goodbye, I pushed the red phone symbol and ended the call.

It took me a few hours to actually laugh about how small minded some people could be. 'Un invitation' it was. I was in shock. Not even at school had I ever been uninvited. Not invited maybe, but uninvited was a whole new experience for me.

How I managed through what I call my "imagine being uninvited to a rugby match" trauma was with a bottle of Prosecco, an Ozzie friend and free to air Channel 10 live match.

Yes, I would be watching the test match live on free to air TV.

This had obviously not occurred to Mae, swooning as she did around the local doctor, as she had invited herself to use his sports channel.

With great delight I sent a text with the full-time result to both Tanya and Mae with a couple of xx timed to coincide with the party kick off and the delayed coverage.

Neither replied.

I chose to continue to say my usual *morena* or *kia ora* when I saw Mae each morning along the corridor, so that she would have to respond although I often caught her shuffling into the waiting room to avoid me.

Don't get mad, get even is my usual style; but I was affronted.

For those who know me, I am an All-Blacks fanatic. When I told my friends they were partially shocked at how weird it was but laughed at me knowing how big a fan I am. All approved of my management of the situation.

The professional relationship was cool between Mae and myself. Interestingly, the other younger nurses and dieticians who also shared the workspace confided and corroborated my opinion of Mae. One of the desert misfits.

At the end of the next week, I was enrolled in a training programme run by external trainers.

When I saw Mae's name on the list, I sighed and wished she wasn't in the group. The programme was Teaching on the Run and I was really looking forward to updating my Adult teaching qualifications. Having Mae on the course could be awkward. It got worse when on the first morning the participant numbers were only four and as there was a lot of sharing and group interaction it was clear we could not avoid each other. I held my smile and she was acting positive too. The memories of my first gush of compliments flooded back, knowing how fake she was, but as the seminar was about teaching and mentoring students, I felt confident I was able to participate in a more engaging manner than she.

Mae's OCD, and what I also suspect is a personality disorder, was evident and she was pushed beyond her self-assured comfort zone. I was encouraging as were the other two participants but my thought bubble was not so gracious, and I was thinking condescending thoughts. Karma was at work. She seemed very much out of her comfort zone. We had a presentation to prepare as homework.

The next day, I arrived at the seminar with my presentation ready. So were two others. Mae wasn't there. One of the facilitators explained that Mae was not able to join as she needed to cover sickness in her GP clinic.

Quick as a flash, Brenda, a colleague manager from ED who was doing the training said. "Really? I know there is no sickness that needs covered, I have just come from the staffing huddle. I don't think she would be able to do the presentation today; that's more likely why she isn't here".

I smiled, but said nothing. I heard through the grapevine (gossip columns of remote nursing) that Tanya got that job, but was attacked by a client and went off sick. She then changed careers to the police force. Mae had a relationship with a nurse who had fled America before going to court to face a charge against her of assaulting an officer in a hospital. She was trying to visit her wife whom she had allegedly assaulted.

There really is never a dull moment when working in a desert. You could never make it up

***

As a midwife, I was afforded the ability to work independently, and we each had our own work space. Up to three midwives provided 24/7 emergency childbirth care, for those whose labours started before they went to either Katherine or Alice Springs for a sit down which is that two weeks pre birthing time when they go to their birthing town. The majority of work was antenatal surveillance and care, which was challenging and time consuming. Postnatal care was provided cooperatively with the child health nurse when the new mothers eventually came back to TC. Sometimes the new babies were met at the supermarket or the bank ATM, and an actual postnatal visit might happen there and then. Always shy, I learned the art of pre-warning them that I needed to ask some women's business questions and these would be asked without eye contact.

We always had a baby car seat in the vehicle and would bring them back to the clinic, then drop them home with their shopping.

The women would know where to come if they had any worries, and the child health nurse kept me informed of their visits for the baby needles. I could meet the new mothers then and have an informal yarn. Contraception was reliably addressed in Alice Springs prior to discharge. Commonly, a contraceptive implant which had its own set of ethical and social ramifications was inserted into their arms and proffered up to three years of contraception.

Although I had not encountered any domestic violence in response to the implants, I had been advised by colleagues and read academic articles discussing the complexities of its use.

25   TENNANT CREEK COMMUNITIES

The Tennant Creek (TC) communities are difficult to describe.

The town itself has a population of about 3000. It has a main street with two café's, three pubs, a memorial club affectionately known as the Memo and a golf course. There is a hardware store and a couple of other generalist stores that the locals call Kmart plus, meaning the goods are bought from Alice Springs Kmart and the plus is the doubling of the price when sold in TC.

There are three petrol stations, one of which has been converted to the supermarket after the IGA was burned down by three preteenage girls last month.

On my first day on the job, I needed to collect a pregnant mum, who had been out of town for sorry business[1]. She was due to go for a sit down in Alice springs.

Google maps might work here but for that, you need to know the correct spelling of streets rather than phonetics and a camp just has numbers. Armed with the verbal directions, I set off to find my first client for the day.

It's hard to know if collecting the young mums and driving them to our clinics is the best thing to do, or not. Some would argue that it takes away their autonomy. What I soon discovered though is that if the women don't want to come with you, they won't. They do have a say. Besides, the camps are all on the outskirts of town and it is a long way to walk when pregnant and in 30-40 degrees heat.

My colleague wished me luck and said don't get out of the car unless you are sure there are no dogs and don't ever go past the gate, because the dogs hide under cars and under the house. Just beep the horn and someone will come out.

As directed, I found the camp and started looking for the number.

Ahead, I could see the settlement as the road narrowed and an oversized speed bump heralded the entrance to town camp. I thought I was prepared for the sight before me, but nothing really can prepare you for something like this.

Each house had space and an outside area of land. There were fridges and washing machines in various states of repair outside. The fences were used to dry clothes. Wheelie bins, litter and broken toys prams and strollers would be strewn across the yard. It was difficult to know if anyone was at home or not.

Most had verandas although some were locked up and abandoned. These were the homes of families who had gone out bush. They would be back. Other family members might move in while they are gone. A five foot wire fence separated each house from their neighbour. Banged-up wrecks of cars are randomly left mostly at the rear of the property. If someone is home there may or may not be a vehicle at the front, most likely a sedan with dings and at least one broken window. I noticed there were no vehicle crossings on the driveways and an absence of 4x4 vehicles. Driving in my NT[2] govt car I felt obscenely conspicuous. A government education vehicle passed me and stopped just ahead; a woman and small child hopped out and went inside.

I continued further into the camp and already I could feel the poverty and smell the inequity. There was a small fire smoking by the concrete water run and a few men walking towards the town. I couldn't find the numbers on the houses. I looked at the gates but there were no letterboxes, hence no numbers. None on the door, nor on the veranda's where mattresses in various states, chairs, clothes in bags and some hanging on bits of rope to dry clothes cluttered every bit of space. The rubbish was stunning in its abundance, and it was everywhere.

Around the first corner was a tidy house with five or six young people sitting on the veranda. I pulled up outside the house and as I did, a young woman came up to the fence.

Two dogs simultaneously charged at the fence. They were light brown, small and skinny, but their bark was terrifying. She yelled at them and people on the porch yelled too. The quiet camp was for a few seconds a screaming yapping insult to the silence.

"Hi, I said. I'm looking for number 21?"

You want Jzata? You the midwife? I smiled, yes. "She over there. First one coming in on that side up there," said the woman. I could sense that the huddle of women had speculated who I was and who I was looking for. I think about confidentiality and how I could never identify myself as the midwife if I was looking for someone's house in London. There are simple concepts of community that do well in remote Australia.

It wasn't until I pulled up outside that house, I noticed the numbers were on the soffit although I have discovered many are no longer there.

I beeped my horn.

A dark black skinned wiry man came out and up to the fence – "I'm looking for Jzata," I said, winding down my window. He waved an acknowledgement, turned quickly and went back inside.

A few minutes later a tall and pregnant woman ambled out. I introduced myself.

Jzata said she was sleepy. Could I come tomorrow, she asked? Of course, I replied at the same time - aye. She turned and disappeared back into the house.

I gave the group at the other house a wave as I passed them on my way out, knowing they had watched every move. They waved back and giggled, showing flashes of white teeth. I thought to myself that they probably all should be at school.

It took three attempts to see Jzata in the clinic and when she eventually did get into the car on Thursday, I told her I was pleased she didn't have dogs because I was scared of them. She thought this was funny. She told me her dogs only bite sometimes. They won't bite you. I'll keep them away, she assured me.

My office at Tennant Creek.

Ornithophobia they call it...and I haven't got it anymore. Or I like to think that .

I had worked hard to overcome the fear I had acquired during my childhood. It was a real fear. I have a scar on my nose to remind me of the now forgotten rooster attack. I was only a wee girl when that happened. But I remembered the seagulls swooping down on me when I was in high school. Not once, but twice. It was horrid. I had to change my route to school because of those fecking seagulls.

But over the years as a mother, I had made a grand effort to calm my ornithophobia so as not to pass it on to my children.

It had worked or so I thought until not that long ago. It happened when I first arrived and was on my way to my first placement in Benalla. A big black and white magpie decided I was too close to her nest. Oh! the sight I must have been - throwing my handbag in the air and screaming like a banshee to protect myself from the horrible bird. And to add insult to injury I got not an ounce of sympathy from my Ozzie colleagues who just laughed and said how lovely magpies are... and did I know they were protected?

Protected me arse. The only good magpie is a dead one.

So now I find myself in the middle of the desert where magpies are less in number – but big black crows - or are they ravens - are now reigniting my fear.

There is one demon who I am eyeing up for a fight. He thinks he is too clever by half. He squawks and keels outside my office window and then I hear a loud tap tap tap tap tap on glass.

The fecker is trying to trip the automatic door to let himself in.

I think I'd die if he did.

As if magpies, crows, and cheeky dogs aren't enough to deal with, I had a close encounter with a Rooster. A client who was living in the hostels in Tennant Creek asked me to pick her up from her dads house and gave me the address. When I arrived I pulled into the drive and got out to say "gidday" to the gathering of people sitting on their verandah. To my horror the Fowl came charging towards me. I jumped into the car. This was very funny for the family to see. The lovely mum giggled and giggled and we would often have a laugh about that day

---

Marisha had just turned nineteen. She was tall, very dark skinned, had fine facial features with white teeth and a bright engaging smile. Like many of the Northern Territory indigenous women, her legs were so thin it was hard to imagine them supporting body weight, and her skinny arms needed a paediatric cuff to get an accurate blood pressure measurement from.

This was how they are built.

They walk slowly to conserve energy in the heat, are always barefooted and seem remarkably healthy.

From behind there was no evidence that she was pregnant and had a healthy size bump of thirty-four weeks when I first met her.

As the third midwife arriving to fill a gap vacant for months, Marisha was allocated to my caseload. She had a positive relationship with my colleague who had been in TC for over a year, and I quickly got to know her. She always came to her appointments and would often ask for a lift home or to one or other homes of her friends. We were encouraged not to be a taxi service, but it was good knowledge to accrue for the times we needed to 'chase the women up'; we would know where to start looking.

Besides, it was a kind thing to do for any pregnant woman.

Marisha was naive as well as beautiful, but unfortunately had learned that alcohol numbed feelings and she was not able to stop drinking, even while pregnant. As a midwife we were on call for obstetric emergencies. During her pregnancy she had many presentations to the Emergency Dept, either having fallen or just being drunk. Each stay would necessitate a midwifery review.

This sweet and troubled young woman would light up when I would peep through the ED curtains. To her, the midwives were on her side. Alcohol had become an escape from her conscious life. She would promise to stop drinking of course. She would apologise. She would reliably wait until we called in to see her when she had sobered up the next morning.

We would take her home.

I learned interesting practices within indigenous culture through Marisha. The father of her baby was from Tennant Creek and so she was expected to live with his family. This was often difficult for young women. It seemed Marisha was not made welcome, and it was more difficult because his family house was next to the reserve where her brother had died by suicide when they were both young kids new to the town. Her own mother was living in Mt Isa, many miles away. She too drank alcohol excessively and so I was witnessing the true impact of Foetal Alcohol Spectrum Disorders also known as FASD.

A FASD child having a baby.

When she had sobered up after one of her frequent visits to the ED, she asked me, "Teresa, is my baby being born at Christmas?"

"Yes, it will be born around that time." I said.

"Is that tomorrow?"

"No Marisha, it is a long time away."

"My cousin said it is Christmas tomorrow."

The look of confusion and disillusionment seemed to pass

through her eyes and over her body. Sadness cloaked her for the briefest of moments.

I realised that Marisha had very limited understanding of time, maybe of anything much in the world of pregnancy and mothering.

Her young partner was often with her and kept telling her not to drink. But these words are empty coming from another drunk.

After one of her binges, Marisha had agreed to go into rehab in Alice Springs and a place was secured for her by the Alcohol and Drug team. The bus ticket was booked, and she would go directly to the bus stop from the hospital in the transport van.

I had checked in with her that morning, and she was ready and waiting to go. Ready and waiting just meant she had her phone and charger. Food for the journey had been ordered and a pack of sandwiches, a Just Juice box and apple were in a plastic bag on the bedside locker.

Marisha went missing as the van was ready to leave the hospital. An S.O.S. call was made to the midwives; as though we could magically find her.

I went to the Emergency Dept and out through the waiting room where another young girl was waiting. I asked her if she knew Marisha? They looked about the same age. This girl was her cousin and said she had seen her going towards town. "I think she is going to the post office to get money," said the young woman.

I wondered how she would know this.

"Are you the midwife" she asked?

"Yes, I am".

"Can I see you? I'll wait outside," she said. And so, another woman was added to our books later that day.

I drove to the post office and there was a van with three women in it.

"Have you seen Marisha?" I asked, hedging my bets that they might know her.

The middle-aged woman told me she was in the post office with her cousin, and she would be out in a minute.

I couldn't wait, or more importantly the Greyhound bus wouldn't wait.

The woman in the car was insistent that Marisha was alright, and they would be out in a minute.

To this day, I am not sure why she didn't want me to go into the post office. I did though, just in time to see a wad of money being passed from Marisha to the woman. Marisha tucked the remaining money into her bra.

It perturbed me, but it is possible that Marisha's cousin had some responsibility or access to her cash card and was getting money out for her to take to Alice Springs.

I didn't ask. I suspected some humbugging of money had happened.

I just asked Marisha if everything was alright?

She said it was.

Marisha left on the bus. The midwifery team and alcohol service had high hopes that she would have a positive rehabilitation and, as planned, stay on to birth her baby.

We would see her after Christmas.

As it happened Marisha stayed in Alice Springs one night and caught the bus back to Tennant Creek the next day.

Syphilis screening is part of every woman's early pregnancy blood tests. When I first worked in WA, back in 2006, it was the first time I had encountered positive results. Whatever the public health initiatives were back then, they have not done a good job. On an estimate of my current caseload 1:5 have been exposed to the disease.

It is seldom straight forward.

Ms M is 19 with her second child. She is indigenous and has a history of ETOH[3] use and drinks during her pregnancy. She has a partner, non indigenous guy in his 50's.

Ms M screened positive for syphilis in early pregnancy and has treatment, as does her new partner, however because she has a temporary break up with the FOB (father of the baby) goes to Adelaide and treatment is interrupted.

Later in the pregnancy she returns to her community and to the partner and screens positive with rising titres.

There is ongoing domestic violence, alcohol use and non engagement with midwifery care.

The FOB has controlling behaviours and it is challenging to ever see Ms M alone; however, a chance opportunity arises and we have a conversation while in the car, waiting for Mr W to get the older child from the house.

Ms M pleads with me not to tell Mr W about the syphilis. I reassure her that I can only speak to her about anything regarding her pregnancy but ask to make some time when Mr W won't be with her.

She agrees to come to the clinic the next morning when Mr W is at work.

He comes anyway. Luckily Mr W gets a call from his work asking him where he is.

When I am alone with Ms M, now 36 weeks pregnant with rising syphilis titres she discloses that she had got back with an old boyfriend (probably the reason for rising titres) that she had left Mr W because he was locking her in her room, not letting her use a phone and throwing things.

Sadly, I was not surprised.

Then she said, "I stole all his money and spent it when I went to Adelaide and now he wants it back."

Two sides to the coin. The plot thickened.

I had seen through the previous midwifery phone correspondence how Mr W had been stalking her on a social media sites and sending the photos to the midwife – telling her what an unfit mother she was.

This was not a typical day as a midwife, but sadly the elements are all so very common. That day Ms M had her first of three double IM injections to treat the syphilis.

I commenced mandatory reporting.

The sexual health nurse would be following up her contacts and who knows the outcome of it all?

She would get to sit down and complete treatment, however her baby when born would be in neonatal for some time.

As for the domestic violence and physical abuse that was disclosed, I have no answer.

***

I was once given the book, "*Alexander and the terrible horrible no good very bad day*" by Judith Viorst & Ray Cruz. At the end of Alexanders' terrible horrible no good very bad day he says, "some days are like that, even in Timbuktu" That sentiment is relevant as a remote midwife.

My compassion tank was nearing the end. As it happened, I was now the only midwife in the town, with a client load of three midwives. One colleague went on long leave but no replacement for the third had arrived. The hospital manager seemed for reasons known only to herself not to be able to tell me when another colleague would start. "its all sorted, don't worry sister" was her patronising reply. This didn't help. I had become wary of staff who stay too long in remote areas. But that's a whole other story.

I had gotten used to my day being full of surprises, changes, drop in opportunistic appointments. This day was very much like that. It started with our Aboriginal liaison officer having two women to collect, one to attend a scan and the other to see me. Both were unable to come to their appointments because they were probably sleeping or in houses behind locked fences.

***

. . .

I got a referral from the indigenous health care of a fourteen year old girl, presenting well into her pregnancy, with a positive STI screen. This would mean we needed to get her into the clinic and give antibiotics to treat the chlamydia and trichomonas infection. A referral to Territory Families as part of mandatory reporting was done. Our ALO couldn't locate the young woman, or do we call her a young child? It's a dilemma on many fronts. When we eventually met, in my attempt to engage her with midwifery services I showed her around our clinic. She was a confident young woman. I explained that simply because of her age, other people from other agencies would need to ask her lots of questions. "I won't tell nobody nothing," she said knowingly and defiantly. This meant she knew how it all worked. That she would have to disclose who the father of the baby was, and if she didn't then at the time of birth, the baby's cord blood would be collected for DNA to eliminate or confirm the father. From then on it was anyone's guess as to what happened - prison was usual. It's horrible.

Trying to keep the communication open, I reassured her by saying that in the clinic room it was all about her and her growing baby. She didn't respond.

All was going reasonably ok, until I went to the ED to get a prescription and dispense antibiotics for her STI. The new doctor insisted on seeing the young woman instead of accepting my midwifery referral. I reiterated that she was fourteen, showed him the laboratory results and suggested it was often best for women to be treated in the privacy of my clinic room.

He insisted he see her in ED. I took her to triage. She didn't stay. I knew she wouldn't.

The doctor at ED said, "well it's all organised for next time." I just said, there might not be a next time... and thought to myself -until she presents in labour again.

***

Ms H was an older mother to be, having her third child; she too had not engaged in care, except for remote management of her now spiralling type 2 diabetes. English was her second or third language, and when I met with her, I found a quiet and shy woman, seemingly keen to engage in her pregnancy but with a gap in the knowledge of the impacts on her diabetes and unborn baby. A challenge for women like Ms H is to access good health care as she and her partner were transient. How long they would be in this community, no one would know.

She needed an eye watering amount of insulin during this pregnancy and I felt the burden of responsibility to coordinate getting a doctor to prescribe the doses, ensure she accessed the insulin pens from the pharmacy, and then knew how to correctly administer. This was an almost impossible task. I called to her address to check her readings for the diabetic remote tele-health for the next morning. I had been to visit her a few times, so the various family members knew who I was.

Ms H lived in a tent at the back of a house in a community. I pulled up in my car and got out.

The two men sitting on the porch said hello. "I'm looking for Ms. H," I said. Another woman came out of the house. I waited outside. The smell from the building was putrid and the heat made it worse. Nappies and rubbish were everywhere. I wonder why or when the poverty and filth happened. I wondered if those living inside these homes knew how unsanitary it was. Too many people lived under too few roofs. There was a local electrician working inside fixing the air con. I wondered what he thought or if was he, like me, getting used to it but not really used to it.

The woman called to a young boy and spoke in language telling him to go out through the hole in the fence to tell Ms H that I was there.

The tall overweight Ms H came out and we yarned[4] and she showed me her blood sugar readings. This was progress. Then she said she didn't have any insulin left.

Fail fail fail. That's what I felt. Despite all the efforts and appointments with indigenous health diabetic educators, pharmacists etc, at the end of the day, this pregnant woman didn't have any insulin left. I sorted it. But it will likely continue to happen.

Back at my clinic Ms M who was overdue for her rheumatic heart prophylaxis didn't make it to her appointment. She lives in a community one hour out of town and phoned to say she would call into antenatal clinic around 2pm. They have no health centre and she is dependent on getting a lift into town for any appointments. I'm not sure when she will be in now.

More phone calls about our new fourteen year old client from Territory Families asking if the client had disclosed who the father of the baby was. As if this was a priority. Not for the midwife. The police and sexual assault team would soon be involved.

Then I got a call from Ms T. She had arrived back in town two days earlier with her newborn son. Ms T had been flown to Alice Springs as her blood pressure was dangerously high and so had been commenced on antihypertensives and magnesium sulphate infusion to prevent pre eclampsia seizures; then fast tracked for delivery.

As she was about to be flown out, she became upset. The doctors in ED had told her that she would most probably have her baby that day, and most probably via caesarean birth. Ms T did not want this. She asked me if this was true.

The medication worked very effectively in lowering her blood pressure. I said this was a good sign, and if her readings were stable and remained so when she got to Alice Springs she would need to talk with the doctors.

As an antenatal educator from way back, empowering women

with the knowledge of how to ask the right questions was integral in women having consent.

I said to Ms T, tell the doctors you do not want to have an operation. Ask the doctors if you have time to think about it; and also ask the doctors if you can have a normal birth.

Maybe the wording was not quite as clinical as that but I tried my best to empower her. I did explain that if the blood pressure didn't stay down then there might not be a choice. She nodded.

Be strong, I said, as she left on the ambulance trolley.

So here she was back with her newborn son, a beautiful little boy, dressed in a wee green baby gown.

I knew she had had a vaginal birth, but I wanted to hear it from her.

"what happened when you got to Alice Springs?" I asked. She beamed the biggest smile.

"They wanted to give me the operation but I said no" She waited for my response.

Wow, how did that feel? I asked. She said, "They told me I had to. Then I asked if I could just wait coz I didn't want an operation. Another doctor came and said it was alright and so I got the needle in my back."

I took this as induction with syntocinon and epidural analgesia.

She had the biggest smile when she told me and was so happy to show off her new son to me.

A small win in what was otherwise a terrible horrible no good very bad day.

26 WA BORDER OPENING

As the Governor of WA opened the borders, for me it was an opening of an opportunity; so I made the quick decision to quit my contract and go back to WA. I was surprisingly homesick and felt isolated in the desert.

As an agency midwife it is not an easy decision. I had loved the work, my office, the women and had gotten to be part of the community. I had helped behind the scenes at the local pub (managed by a Kiwi of course) with a game evening. This was not a games evening with pub quiz and bingo, that I had thought I had offered to help with but a feast of game and matched wine. I got to taste crocodile and emu, kangaroo, barramundi, rabbit and camel. I had many a good yarn with Fabian who was on a travel visa from Norway, who took his barista skills to Fremantle: a small and smaller world opened when he was serving coffee at my local coffee shop a few months later. I met a gaggle of teachers and we spent many evenings watching the sun setting from the only hill within miles. But the window had opened. Covid was thick in the UK, so I knew I would need to stay a while longer, but I needed to go to Whānau[1]. So, the prep for leaving began.

The BMW had served me well, but I needed new front tyres. It is a European vehicle. The tyres were not stock standard and needed to be ordered in. With the Covid delays, I would be cutting it fine, but they arrived in time. There was a problem though. The Tennant Creek tyre shop did not have the tool bit to extrapolate the nuts off the tyres to change them. They were anti-theft nuts! My BMW became the talk of the town as the lads tried every bloke shop or avenue to procure the bit. As luck would have it, special nuts were found by accident in one of the outdoors shops and after stripping off the original and changing the tyres, these new nuts were screwed back on.

The tyres ended up costing a fortune and now I had the additional dilemma of having no way to change either back tyre should I get a puncture. Ignorance is bliss sometimes. I had travelled 6000 km across Australia by myself. If I had had the misfortune to have punctured a tyre then I would have been completely buggered and at the mercy of the occasional truckie. I had no idea that one very small piece of kit could cause so much chaos. But now that I knew, I was slightly anxious to say the least. All I needed to do was make it to Kununnara. They would surely have the special European size bit.

I called in to buy a sun shade for my car. My reputation had preceded me. When I said that I wanted it to fit my BMW, the man said " oh you are the Kiwi midwife with the BMW?"

A little taken aback I said, "how do you know?"

"Ah!" he said, "Tony came looking for three wheel nuts and by chance I had a few. It was your lucky day," he said.

"Have you got anymore left?" I asked. "I still have the back wheels to rescue."

" I have indeed." he went and bought out eight wheel nuts. "They're all yours, I was going to throw them out."

"You are pretty epic driving all that way by yourself," he said.

I had heard this a lot, but didn't really think it was anything special.

. . .

As it happened, I managed to get to Kununurra and found the one motor business that could change the nuts on the rear wheels.

I never did get a flat tyre the whole trip.

Just before Kununurra, I was stopped by another Covid border patrol. I had forgotten about these, but had my G2G, (good to go) pass that allowed me to cross into Western Australia.

I had my border check first. The WA cop was a young officer and I recognised his pommie accent.

"What part of old blighty are you from?" I asked.

"A place called Bury St Edmonds" he said, it's not far from London."

"Oh my daughter, Hannah has just built a house there," I said. We chatted easily then and my pass was checked and ticked and recorded in some cyber place. I felt nice and happy that I had been able to chat with this policeman. He too was finding the Covid isolation difficult and his parents had been planning to come out for a visit but hadn't been able to travel. We had a shared nod. Back at the border, the fruit quarantine officer started his form.

No, I didn't have any fruit, yes I did have a chilly bin. He had to check it, and also he needed to check the boot.

Shit! The boot!

He saw my hesitation and had a worried look.

"Well," I said. "There's a story with the boot. It's just that the boot latch broke and my mechanic in TC has done a MacGiver with a piece of wire and he said he wasn't sure if it would close after I opened it next time.

"So..," I continued having the full attention of the officer.

"How about we do a deal? I'll open it so long as you help me close it if it breaks again."

"Here – I've got the bungee cords already in case I need them."

He looked at me and said, "You haven't got any fruit, have you"

"Nope." I said "I promise I haven't – the boot is full of my worldly possessions, and I don't plan to open it until I make it to Bunbury."

"Ah well – you're right to go then," he said.

Imagine if I was a drug mule, I thought but dared not say it out loud.

In 2006, I worked on a contract in Kununurra, but my memories of the place were vague. As I drove down the main street, I didn't even recognise the Coles supermarket where I had been called a white ***t. I was shocked at the time, but now I don't blink an eye. Living in the Northern Territory many of the locals have disempowered the derogatory word and have a bumper sticker CUintheNT. However, I did recall the fascinating boat trip I took up the Ord river, where I was weirdly fascinated by the bat trees. I also remembered my exploratory trip to Wyndham on the day Steve Irwin died from a stingray attack.

It was in Kununurra that I first encountered patient-controlled epidural technology, which was a prototype with a simple bag of premixed medication and a syringe refill system that worked well. However, I imagine the cost has now gone up as technology has superseded this. Due to low birthing numbers, I was also the nurse for women.

I left the town to head for Halls Creek, eager to get to my next stop before dark. I borrowed my brother's car for the journey, and he had lived in Halls Creek for over twenty years. We and others called it "Hells Crack," which, like Tennant Creek, had an unfortunate reputation.

Many say the best thing about Hells Crack is the road out. Like my brother, many of us do our utmost best. Sadly it is never enough.

From there, I would drive across to Broome, where my cousin was waiting for a cold glass of Prosecco.

. . .

The familiar termite mounds were dotted across the landscape as I was travelling through the stunning Kimberley's, a vast remote and popular outback venture retreat in Northwest, WA and a mere three times the size of the UK (for perspective). Ahead I I noted the turn off to the Purnululu *Bungle bungles* where my, now adult, sons had had their first tastes of outback camping. Their uncle took them on an adventure, and I remember being terrified that they might be bitten by a snake. Both have magical memories of this trip. It wasn't until I went camping there the following year that I understood their fascination for the place.

Vinny was about ten at the time. He took a photo of an abandoned, (now vintage) car, set against the orange and black layered sandstone domes stretching as far as they could see, and rising high above the spinifex^2 covered plains that surrounds them. A stunning amateur snap, it had recently been used in an RTE (Irish national television) movie trailer.

I sent him a message with the photo of the road sign.

When I arrived at the Halls Creek Hotel, I was warned that to avoid my car being broken into I should park as close to the CCTV as I could and that the gates to the hotel would close at 10pm. The next morning I did a drive by where my brothers house was before I left.

A bit further on, I sped past the turn off to Wolf Creek crater. The magnificent example of a fifty thousand tonne meteorite that landed 300,000 years ago is dwarfed in my mind by the memory of that terrifying psychological thriller's portrayal of the kidnapping and torture of two English backpackers, which was filmed at this location. The place has an eerie feel even to this day. The fact that I was 3000km away did not deter me from checking my rear view mirror a little more often.

Lunch and petrol stop would be Fitzroy Crossing where I had an assignment.

My midwifery buddy, Michelle who was happily living on a narrowboat close to London, had asked me to "look out for Delilah," if I went through Fitzroy Crossing.

I chuckled at this request, firstly because there is only one road (sealed) up here and secondly, how old do dogs grow to??? My plan was to take a photo of any dog in FX and send to her just for a giggle.

Back in 2007, camp dogs were neglected, flea ridden, hungry and unpredictable. Michelle had found Delilah with her prolapsed uterus feeding her pups cowering under the flood prevention stilts of her house. An animal lover to her core, Michelle had taken the dog to the vet and nursed her back to good health and was rewarded with the dog love, which camp dogs are renowned for. It is politically incorrect to call these mutts camp dogs in 2020. They are now known as cheeky dogs, vulnerable yet blameless for their plight around the outback communities. I did a wee tiki tour of Fitzroy crossing and sadly yet gladly there were no "cheeky dogs" to be seen. The veterinary service had done a good job of castrating. Not a descendent of Delilah to be seen. No photo opportunity to send back to London.

My day half travelled, I was acutely aware of the niggle that the town of Derby was presenting.

I had had my first outback midwifery job in 2006. I was a relatively new graduate full of knowledge, confidence and in desperate need of sunshine, having lived in Ireland for three years. Two of my siblings who are West Australian residents were full of enthusiasm for me to have an Ozzie outback adventure.

An opportunity to work with women from Aboriginal cultures held a very strong pull.

With a round of paperwork submitted, proving who I was and that I was apparently competent, we as a family had been on the move again, packing up our Irish dream and heading into a land of opportunity.

This rural outback town hundreds of miles from everywhere was to be my outback debut. Dusty and dry. A tired town that wore the memory of better days and hope of a better future.

It had been thirteen years since I'd been in Derby, having left with precise certainty that I would never ever go back. But here I was TC (thanks Covid). I went to revisit some old ghosts, and recall life-changing memories.

I had a treasured piece of art that had hung on my wall in Highgate. I loved to tell its story. Cassia who was in very early labour came to see me. " Can I have my baby now, sister?"

"You will have your baby soon, but not for a little while," I replied.

" Would you paint me one of your pictures?"

"Womens business?" I asked.

Cassia is from the peoples of north west Kimberley region who are able to create this art. It is sometimes called Bradshaws or Gwion figures.

This would give her a focus other than getting her baby born. And it worked. Two hours later Cassie arrived back with two paintings, of which I chose one and she went on to birth her beautiful baby.

Years later I did meet up with her again. It was a very humbling and emotional rendezvous. I was stunned that she remembered me. Her art is now on my wall in Aotearoa.

Driving past the old hospital and through the town I remembered an Aboriginal woman who came into the unit where I was on midwifery shift. "I've got a terrible cough, sister and a pain in my guts."

Within a short time of her arrival, Shania coughed so hard a wee tiny and fragile baby popped out. None of us expected this. I don't know if Shania knew she was pregnant, but I could only speculate that she did since she had come to the antenatal door and not the ED one. But I won't ever know. What I learned that day and the days following this untimely birth, has carved its way into my midwifery *wairua* (spiritual core)and left a permanent tattoo.

A small team, midwife, doctor and nurse spent hours with this new little life, willing her to breathe and stabilise . I learned the skill of intubation, inflation, cannulation, stabilisation and negotiation team work and as her little body shut down to a world she would never know, I experienced the power of aboriginal women.

Shania sat outside the resuscitation room. This was where she was comfortable. The windows of the nursery meant we knew she was there and she knew we were there too. It was where she felt safe – close by, but not with her tot. My western model of midwifery was conflicted as I knew she had yet to cradle her baby.

The hours went by. Shania sat and waited. She was alone when she presented. No phone. No one to call – she had said she would tell her husband later where she was. He was with the children. Can we call anyone? No they are all out bush she said. Shania was not from the town but from a community a long way away. She sat. "I'll be alright here," she reassured me.

We knew our little charge was not going to make it. The RFDS knew as well and our regular updates and guidance was full of hopeful, yet realistic expectations. With hindsight, I think we tried too long. It's a call that is made as a team. The RFDS were clinical and compassionate. If you can stabilise her, we will send a plane and retrieval team. They waited.

Before we "called it" I went to talk with Shania to see if she would like to be with her baby as she passed.

I was speechless. Until this time, Shania was a woman from out of town, sitting alone outside a resus room; now she was surrounded by her countrywomen. To me it was unbelievable. Busy with the baby, I had heard nothing nor seen anyone arrive. There were eight or nine women who sat in comfortable contemplative silence, not talking nor making any fuss. They were with women. They were the true midwives that day.

Yes, she whispered keeping her gaze downward.

I wrapped baby girl who was still struggling to breathe in a beautiful baby pink wrap and Shania's arms cradled her as she calmed her breath and her child passed into the arms of the ancestors.

Tears escaped in silence.

None of the women who arrived knew Shania. No one had been contacted. It wasn't until after this baby's passing that Shania went into my office to call her husband. She talked in language. Her tears had stopped.

I don't know how the women knew to come? Slowly, they left just as they had arrived.

The next day Shania was due for her antibiotics but nowhere to be seen.

I found her in the lazy boy chair of the birthing room, sitting quietly keeping a young aboriginal woman company while she laboured her first birth.

I was privy to something special that day. It is these moments that keep me being a midwife and keep wanting to be with the indigenous women. They are my teachers.

Seeing the streets, after so many years, I failed to remember much of the goodness that undoubtedly was. I sat for a while near the gate of the nurses' quarters where Michelle and I lived on my second contract to Derby. It was here she had first smelled the aboriginal smell, a putrid mix of oil, body odour and hot sweat that a passerby left in his wake. She had rather dramatically held the smell in her mouth refusing to inhale or swallow it and ceremoniously spat it behind the fence.

Unbeknownst to her, I was quietly crumbling with the weight of a distasteful domestic based phone call.

Later that day, it had been a finger-snap decision to quit our contracts. It required an Oscar performance from Michelle and with the urgency born of desperation, to catch the once-a-week plane, we were gone.

Many moons later, the town had not managed to achieve better days. Woolworths, where my sons had worked with Reg from fruit and Veg, was tatty. The car park where I had first witnessed the rain-soaked bodies of locals feeling the first of wet season was part full, the gift shop had closed and the mural on the outside of the antenatal clinic wall was faded and tagged.

I took a walk to the end of the wharf and laid to rest some domestic skeletons of my time there, and decided the beautiful lessons from the women far outweighed the old bones.

This time I think it really is the last time I will be in Derby.

Prosecco and Whānau were waiting. The reliable sunset on Cable beach and the bubbles that I associate with my European life were a welcome distraction to what was happening to the world and why I was still in Australia.

The journey south through to Perth was inspiring and peaceful.

I had secured a contract in Carnarvon, but by the time I had actually left the NT, I had decided not to take it. The exhaustion and energy required to start afresh had descended upon me and I decided to stay with my siblings and work a bit in the city. I drove through Carnarvon, but didn't call into the hospital. A nice enough wee town, but I was glad to be going to Perth. Along the way, I called into Northampton and that set me off, pining for my former life, not for the first time and neither the last, but to see the town that was named after the town where my boat was moored, was hard. The closer I got to my sisters, the closer the tears were from escaping.

I was mentally drained. I needed to replenish my *wairua* (spiritual energy)

I found refuge. Again. With my siblings.

27 WEALTH

Mainland Australia is the world's largest island but also the smallest continent. The country is divided into six states and two territories. Western Australia WA, the largest state, wants independence.

Apparently, their economy has all the elements (pun intended), to be sustainable and although I have little knowledge of how Australia was carved up politically, coming back to the west and her capital certainly feels different.

I had had a week's down time and was heading north again to start a contract in Carnarvon, the banana capital of Australia. Guilt had gotten the better of me and I negotiated to cover the X'mas and New Year holiday time.

Driving from Fremantle towards Perth CBD, it could be any of Australia's other major cities - modern high-rise office blocks, blue skies and homes facing the water, yachts and floating restaurants - until you see the skyline is dominated by Rio Tinto HQ, showing who runs WA.

Further evidence is demonstrated more clearly as the balance of FIFO -Fly In Fly Out- workers outweighs domestic travellers in the departure lounge. They are predominantly male, of mixed culture yet uniform with their high viz clothing, backpack and stoical acceptance of the Covid processing as they check-in. They have been home for the Fly Out days off and are lining up for the Fly In return to the mines. Amongst the blokes in the queues will be geologists, economists, health and safety managers, cooks, cleaners and truck drivers – the muscley blokes with big bellies. The trucks they manoeuvre have wheels which are a whopping thirteen feet tall; yet, it is deemed a sedentary occupation.

Rio Tinto signage around the airport asks their staff to '*stop the spread*', compulsory screening by gate 6 - *no form no fly*. In the Northern Territory (NT), stopping the spread of Covid was motivated to protect the aboriginal communities. Somehow, I don't think Rio Tinto are doing the same. Earlier this year, the mining giant mined Juukan rock cave sites "by mistake". They apparently knew for over six years that these cave sites were amongst the oldest in Australia, with evidence of continuous human habitation going back 46,000 years. Like the traditional owners of the land, anthropologists and archaeologists, Rio Tinto knew they were sitting on a gold mine.

Different gold mines to different people.

When I take an Uber in London, it's my antipodean accent that is the conversation catalyst. I have to work a little harder down under, but in any hemisphere when a Kiwi and an Sri Lankan are in a cab, the conversation will easily turn to cricket. My knowledge is usually limited to who is playing, if there is a tournament on, and a couple of names of past Kiwi greats or perhaps the latest star. My knowledge today as I made my way to the airport, was that NZ were playing in a test against the Windies in New Zealand. Mr Uber Perth is Sri Lankan so the chat easily moved on to how great Kaine Williamson is. By nodding and agreeing I find I don't have to know much more as the drivers spiel off stats and incidentals - just happy to be talking cricket.

My all-time record was in the taxi to Singapore Airport on my journey to Australia back in November BC (before covid) and the day before the Rugby World cup final in 2019. During the chit chat of introductions, having disclosed he (the cab driver) was from Sri Lanka, I had hedged my bets and rather than talk cricket, just said I lived next door to Brian McKechnie. Mr Uber Singapore knew all about the infamous " underarm match" against Australia in 1981 and I got to hear his version of it. The entire journey to the airport was a one way conversation that seemed to give him a delightful distraction. I'm sure Mr Uber Singapore would have known McKechnie was also an All-Black but that conversation would have to be another day.

Mr Uber Perth was, however, curious about where I was flying to today. Covid had changed the face of travel and he was happy to hear I was a midwife going to Carnarvon. My wife is a doctor he said, we lived in Derby for four years. And so the cricket conversation took a swift turn to health in the Kimberley's – there was enough common ground - we both had lived in Derby. I said I was there last week. That was a shock to him! I didn't share my thoughts of how tired the town was now; we both just talked about the people we still knew in common, the harsh school environment and the magnificent sunsets.

WA may be the biggest state in Australia, but the world is still small.

28 CANARVON

This was my shortest contract. Four weeks which incorporated Christmas and New Year. I did not have any births, and very few postnatal women and babies to care for. Our Christmas Eve born baby was as close to a Christmas baby as could be. I bought the mother and her wee baby a gift to have at the end of the cot. I think she was shocked. The new mum certainly smiled when she found the gifts.

And then there was Ted, the only other patient on the ward. Ted could have gone home but decided to stay with us. Ninety three years young, he was from a plantation and was a dapper old man. I got him a shiny bar of chocolate, so he too could open something on the day. He had Christmas lunch with us. But what a miserable excuse of a meal. I think Carnarvon takes the prize for stingy Christmas staff dinner. My meal delivered at 10:30 was two supermarket slices of ham, one roast potato, pumpkin and some peas. Shockingly mean. But what saved the day was one of our staff, who had obviously known what a disaster Christmas dinner on shift would be, had cooked up a feast of Indonesian food. So Carnarvon has a reprieve.

My one regret was that I didn't have a vehicle while I was there, and I have decided now that I will never go to any placement without wheels.

Working and living with strangers can be the biggest challenge as a midwife and knowing that you can just up and go for a tiki tour at any time, for me, is a sanity saver.

It was a delightful month. My accommodation was in a Renal unit accommodation block that was not used. The single bed was my only complaint, it was brand new and had lovely living and kitchen facilities and was a stone's throw from the hospital.

In my one month there, I met Catherine who was in a new relationship with Kaine, a good looking Māori gentleman from Sydney. Catherine and Kaine were a refreshing and good souled couple. They had met online and both had been married twice. It was clear to me that they fit.

Catherine was a brave and inspiring woman. She had suffered personal loss that as a mother no one should do, so was on a healing journey. Kaine and she met at the perfect time.

They stayed with me at Fremantle and visited when I was in Fitzroy Crossing, bringing in supplies of NZ wine to keep me sane. Regretfully, when it was our turn to visit them while we were on our road trip later in the year, the community of Nhulunbuy was closed due to an outbreak of Covid in Darwin.

Not long after I left Carnarvon, Catherine and her Kiwi love match also left their jobs, continuing their adventures across the state. She sent me a photo of Kaine serenading her on some remote beach. This lovely couple had eloped.

Good things happen in that wee town.

Midwifery services in Rural Australia are in constant struggle to meet the needs of their indigenous populations to birth on country and cater to the non indigenous Australians and those of immigrant families. There continues to be a constant struggle to retain staff and keep the services open. Simple services like antenatal education are not reliably available so when I met a couple in the antenatal clinic who were desperate to learn hypno-birthing, for her second baby's birth at the end of January, I was so happy to be able to teach this skill.

The next evening the soon-to-be father picked me up and took me to their home on a mango plantation.

We had a three hour session in hypno-birthing and I was sent home with a bag full of the most delicious mangoes. What a pleasure that was! The mum had to relocate to a tertiary centre for their birth so we met for a refresher over a coffee at Mosman Park in Perth. During this time, she was able to reflect and decide what she wanted for her birth and made her decision to go back to Carnarvon to birth her second child.

Baby M was born on her due date in Carnarvon with the lovely midwives by her side. Now whenever I eat a mango, I always offer up a thought to this family.

29 METRO MIDWIFE IN PERTH

Completing paperwork and online competencies is tiresome. I'm of the opinion that we as a profession have more boxes ticked as competent, yet less practical, ability. I doubt if anyone is actually bothering to check if I wash my hands correctly or don or doff my PPE in the correct order; but each time I've moved to a new hospital or interstate, I've demonstrated that I'm competent to do so. Drug calculations, managing emergencies, and basic life support are all tick-boxed. The reality is that I will seldom encounter some tasks, and even though my competency register is completed, if I don't know how to do something, I won't do it until I check the right way.

Management of emergencies and complex situations is relatively rare, and it is essential that we have drills to refresh, but ticking boxes doesn't make me competent.

Every day, every shift, a midwife hopes doing our best is enough.

It hit the news this week (January 2021) here in Australia, that a mother in a private hospital south of Perth was given ten times more morphine than the correct dose. The hospital has stated the staff involved have been stood down/resigned, and the parents have gone public to tell their stories. The mother was in a coma, suffered a cardiac arrest, and has recovered, but their precious baby boy died.

I don't know the situation nor am I commenting on this tragedy, but I've come to know that midwives are losing their voice and skill. By no means is it a deliberate cause and effect but having spent the last year working in four remote hospitals, midwifery has become medicalised, and the midwifery voice is now a whisper.

I will be following this case to find out what happened. How does this kind of error occur?

Perhaps we will learn that the midwifery voice has stopped the midwife from speaking.

I worked my first shifts in Metro Perth last weekend. At 5 am a phone call lifted me from my sleep, and I SatNaved my way across the city. Postnatal care principles are universally unchanged, the demographics of the mothers certainly have, and the implications of mode of delivery, i.e. increased vacuum and caesarean section births.

Not a new phenomenon by any means, but I noticed some medicalisation and changes to care. Some of the changes are good, even though they are in response to iatrogenic factors. One example is bladder care. Each state in Australia has different policies and clinical indicators to manage this. I asked a colleague on my first shift about their management, and she told me that anyone who has a first void of > 700 mls needs an in-out catheter. Oh really? Yes, she said, we have had a few overstretched bladders, so now everyone has to have a catheter reinserted for 24 hrs. And so it goes on. My point is not about bladder care per se; it is about midwives just doing what they are told and not making any critical patient-centered thinking.

Having said this, not thinking and just doing is the new normal because of patient load. At the hospital, I first did my agency shifts. The allocation is supposed to be 5 clients to 1 midwife (a mother and baby equate to one). Add one more client and it becomes 6 : 1 or 12:1 counting the babies. Each mother and baby have a bedside chart for obstetric and care plans, and each has progress notes. All in all, one mother and one baby has four places that need documented care each shift. Having six patients - if my maths are correct - in one 7hr shift, I needed to document 24 files.

I have a competency in drug calculations, so I hope I got that one right.

So, not thinking becomes a way to survive as a midwife. By not thinking, we lose our voice. When we lose our voice, we don't know how to notice something is not quite right.

Every midwife around the world will want to know what happened in this recent case. I'm hedging my bets that human error and system failure will both play a part.

***

Over the years, I've danced with many varying thoughts and judgments about Private v/s Public maternity care.

I was very 'judgy' until I was a student midwife in Limerick.

It's seldom we were allocated to the Private rooms, and as students did a lot of piss taking of the midwives who, in our minds, fussed and bustled around the private patients (PP).

One morning, I was allocated to prepare a PP for her elective caesarean(c/s). Handover was Mrs. W in room 1, one of Dr. R's private patients.

I still held the opinion that it was strange to elect a c/s but I was mature enough not to question the client, especially on the day of surgery.

Her room was the first inside the door of the M1 ground floor postnatal ward. As I prepared this first-time mother, I went through the standard checklist, ticking and giving little snippets of advice.

I looked at this 23 year old slim beautiful young woman in front of me and said to her, "Your surgery line will be about this long, demonstrating with my thumb and forefinger outstretched, and it will be so low you will still be able to get into your bikini, and it won't be seen."

She looked at me and said, "I don't worry about scars; my body is covered in them."

Oh! I mentally scanned what I could see of exposed skin, wondering if perhaps she had tattoos removed, which seemed to be a 'thing' at the moment.

"What are your scars from?"

I had Hodgkin's lymphoma when I was eighteen and relapsed, so I've got scars and marks everywhere.

What a slap in my face this was. Firstly, annoyed at not being given an appropriate handover, and secondly, shock and relief I had not mentioned what was in my mind.

I had one of Oprah's *ah haa* moments.

That lovely woman started me on a personal journey of self-reflection. Firstly, as in life, you never know what has gone on before you met this person. Secondly, woman-centered care is that. Until this time, I had thought I was providing women-centred care by way of convincing and presenting the choices that I thought were 'best for women.' Now I put aside my beliefs and feel I'm a true fence sitter. I miss being that midwife who always believed that natural, calm, incense-filled birth is the best way. I still have many colleagues and friends who fit this bill and fill the shoes.

In any handover, it is pretty standard to hear private, biased, judgmental statements.

Even as recently as last Christmas, I was pre-warned that our only patient in Carnarvon was "acting like a private patient," "bit of a princess."

I told my Limerick story that day.

On another private v/s public note, I worked a shift in a Perth Metro facilities that are both private and public. This seems to be a common business health model. I imagine following the American system.

This shift was in the SCBU - Special Care Baby Unit. Aside

from getting the bitchface welcome from one of the permanent staff, I had four wee feeding and growing babies to care for and got on with the shift.

The mother of twins I was allocated to, had decided to start pumping her milk to feed them, so I got the kit and kaboodle and pulled the curtains to afford her some privacy as she started expressing.

A bitch-faced colleague threw herself past the curtains, about to berate the mother, stopping only when she saw me.

"Oh, you are here. Then it's alright. We are not allowed to pull the curtains."

This bitchface had already questioned me on miserably minor issues. This happens to agency staff at times. Some resent the freedom and higher pay rates that agency staff get. It happens all over the world.

As I was supervising this mum with her first pumping, I just smiled and said, "Oh, thanks," not showing my utter disbelief that I couldn't pull curtains in an open ward.

After this, I noticed the curtains around each bay where the babies were all tucked up in their bassinets.

They were beautiful, child-friendly colours, in very good condition, non-permanent fabric, and all neatly Velcroed out of the way, some actually tucked up and over the railing.

At the change of shift, I asked my colleague, "Whats the story with the curtains – I got told off for pulling them around earlier."

This was her reply.

"Oh, we are not allowed to use them. They are here for decoration. It's because we are both private and public. So private governance means we have to have curtains, but public rules are that we are not allowed to use curtains ever since that baby died in Bunbury."

"What?" I asked.

"Oh, there was a seventeen year old father who threw a baby, and no one saw it because the curtains were closed."

"So it was the curtain's fault?" I said, incredulous.

She laughed – "Yeah, ridiculous isn't it?"

"So what about privacy for any of our mums?" "Oh, we encourage the mums to turn their chairs, so their backs are facing out."

"And the Muslim mums?" I asked, and, as I said it, wondered if I had seen many Muslims in Perth.

"Oh, she replied, they can feed their babies under the shrouds."

I didn't have the words to respond to this statement. I just cringed, and as it was time to go home, I did exactly that.

They asked me if I would like to work the next day. I booked my second shift.

30 DID THAT JUST HAPPEN?

There is a shortage of midwives in Australia. Most likely, there is a shortage worldwide. I, however, have a caveat on my midwifery employment status. I don't work in the delivery suite, and I don't do night duty. When the shutters closed on my Aotearoa holiday on 14 March, 2020 and London went into lockdown for the first time, I delivered my last baby.

It was both memorable and poignant as my phone entered a state of hyperactivity unknown prior to coronavirus, I glimpsed at the text from my lovely daughter, who was about to tidy off her sofa for her mother's visit, it simply said, "Mum, I don't think you can come." I took a deep breath and refocused on the wonderful woman who was birthing her third child in the rural town hospital in Victoria. A beautiful, calm, gentle birth unfolded as the world went into chaos. I was happy knowing this was most likely my last birth. I had no idea what the world was going to throw at me, but I decided that I would no longer pander to the stress of birthing women and that night duty could take a flying fuck.

A year on, I find myself again accidentally in Perth, working for the agency that has just featured in the national news because one of the doctors (I assume they are paying megabucks to), didn't read the fucking instructions and overdosed two elderly folks with the life-saving Covid vaccine. The agency is huge and about to take a skate, I presume? I worked with them on my first round of sunshine seeking when I was a newly qualified midwife. Only the paperwork has changed. And the workload.

I have one very vivid memory of working for this agency then. It was my first foray into private midwifery. I hated having to charge for every syringe or sanitary pad I gave out, but I loved that the women were treated as princesses and had double beds even for the women having caesarean births. It took me a while to get used to half-naked men wandering about the room in the early morning. I think I would secretly like it now. What I remember most vividly was the room's views, a sweeping float of the Swan river with the black-feathered birds of the same name idly doing what swans do, swanning around.

I have taken this blissful memory to my midwifery colleagues all around the world, overestimating just how delicious private midwifery care can be. The Ozzies did it right, I would say. I told my London manager this too. In arguably the poshest hospital in Europe, they never did get double beds. In fact, I remember the day the one and only double bed disappeared. Gone. No explanation. No discussion. Gone. It was popular. But not with the clients from countries afar.

So when I returned many years later as an agency midwife to my Utopic postnatal ward, my bubble burst. Unrecognisable, but for the view. That, too, had changed with a stadium on the banks, but the Avarian families still lived there, and the calm vista remained.

The call had come in firstly to cancel one shift, so I blissfully snuggled into the pillow only to get another call offering a seven hour postnatal shift. I did the mental acrobatics of, "will I? won't I? Oh fuck it, think of the money" and said yes. Before I could think too much about it, I was driving into the rising sun and ready for my 7am start.

When the staff in the hospital uniforms greet an agency midwife with absolute relief, rather than envy tinctured disdain - which is more usual - you know it is going to be a busy shift.

And it was. Perhaps the most patient-overloaded, staff-deficient shift I've ever done. I felt so sorry for the women and my colleagues, who were all so very kind - again unusual, to be honest – that I said yes to continuing for a twelve hour stint. They literally had a ward full of new mums, brand new babies, and nervous fathers. They had one midwife and an enrolled nurse for over 23 patients.

I hate to hark back to the good old days when this private facility was a dream, but we provided excellent care – we had phones, the women could call us directly instead of pushing a button with the emoticon of an air hostess, and our allocation was four mums and babies. This particular Saturday, I had a staggering seven for the first half, and then it was "team care," meaning it's a free for all. Because documentation in midwifery is more important than care nowadays, each mother and baby have four files – two each, surprisingly enough. So even though maths was never my strong point, I had to clearly and contemporaneously document in 28 files. 28 files! The documentation in health has gone crazy. But 'Jo Bloggs' has signed up for it for litigation. I scream to whoever will listen. If we documented less, we could care more. Document more and care less. Rant over for now. I clocked up 15000 steps that day, felt as though I had not provided adequate care, and my bubble had well and truly burst. This is a healthcare facility gone wrong.

By about 1600 hours, I was tired. My bladder hurt. My feet were sore. There were three of us working with an in-charge appearing from time to time to apologise and disappear back to the labour ward.

I was checking out a drug with Eileen, who, as an Enrolled nurse, had never worked in Maternity when the emergency bell went. Instantly, forgetting my full bladder and sore feet, I went to where the alarm was going, assuming that it would be a "Oops, sorry I pushed the wrong bell," but there was a woman bearing down, making the unmistakable whole woman noises of a female about to give birth. I grabbed some gloves, and my hands went to where a baby was about to fly from. The young Irish midwife who I hadn't seen before, yelled for someone to get a delivery pack. We motioned the woman onto her side on the bed as a meconium-filled bag of membranes emerged.

"Call the paeds please," I heard my automated voice call as I gently protected the woman's perineum and the baby's head slipped to the outside. I watched, and with the wonder I never get used to, saw restitution - the little life turn and spiral through his mother's pelvis, stunned but in good condition, and placed him onto his mother"s tummy.

A towel appeared from somewhere, and he was dried and his healthy transition was complete. Then an old fogey of a midwife lorded over the proceedings with a "Dry that baby for god sake, here," as she rubbed the new little person to within a hair of his life, or so it seemed. There are always those midwives around. I'm glad I'm not one of them. This little fellow was doing grand.

Then a blond woman in her forties with a long severe face, too much makeup, and hoop earrings appeared at the bedside. A boy dressed in black jeans, a singlet, t-shirt, and ears full of rings was hovering behind.

What unfolded haunts me to this day. The new mum's first words were, "I'm sorry, I tried to stop. I'm sorry, I'm sorry, I'm sorry."

"What the fuck's going on?" said the woman.

I intervened. "It's all ok; the baby is fine."

"It's not ok. This is my first grandchild. I'm the grandmother, and I wasn't even here." She left my stare and turned to the bed directing her poison to the woman who had just laboured and birthed a wee baby. The boy, who I assumed to be the son of the bitch, and father of the child, was in shock, but was following the energy of his mother and instead of giving a reassuring kind word, just said, "We were here, why didn't you call me?"

I think that if I could have, I would have figuratively slapped both of these imbeciles. Instantly, I was aware that the room was full of obstetric and paediatric staff, so instead I told the new father in no uncertain terms to go and bond with his baby - NOW. "He's over there", I declared, – stating the obvious. The baby was with the paeds team on the recussitare.

The rhetoric continued from the mouth of the grandmother. "Enough," I said louder than I intended, but I was so annoyed at her.

"Go and look at your grandson", I continued as the young mother cried and snotted, "Sorry, sorry, sorry. I tried, I really did. I put my legs together, but it just came out. I'm sorry."

And so it was. My calm, gentle birth in Benella was not the last one I was to deliver. I accidentally delivered a poor innocent into a farm.

Meanwhile, the medical brigade had arrived. A young doctor leaned into the birthing space and yanked on the umbilical cord.

"Oi," I said. Leave it! She hasn't had any ecbolic yet; it's a physiological third stage.

"How about we transfer around to labour ward?" We did just that, and as we entered the labour room, I took my gloves off and said to the young Irish midwife, "All yours, I have got the whole ward to look after."

With meconium liquor and blood on my shoes and down my work pants, I wiped them clean with alcohol wipes, washed my hands, and went back to the ward at the end of the shift. The memorable, horrible, accidentally overloaded, under cared midwifery shift.

The Ozzies have lost their edge.

31 STILL STUCK IN AUSTRALIA

My next venture was back in the Kimberley's, the northwest of Western Australia. This time as a Community Midwife. My philosophy of "be careful about what you wish for" again has shown that if you are meant to have your wish, it will happen.

I was on my sojourn, house-sitting up to my eyeballs, reading about Irish Antenatal policies and governmental initiatives, when my wish was heard by the universe. My midwifery colleagues, where I had trained in the west of Ireland, had spotted a job that they knew I would love. So I applied and embarked on the task of preparing for the Irish job interview system and remembering the challenge that this would present.

When my mobile rang, I was relieved to take a distraction from the policies and answer the unknown caller. A plucky and familiar Cork accent greeted me. Roisin was making a cold call from her recruitment office in Sydney with the offer of work opportunities in WA. I've had many such calls and answered, "Well thanks, but I'm in Perth and with an agency already. I added to Roisin, I'm actually applying for a job in Ireland. Before long, I had exchanged my Irish connections with an invite to visit her family on the remote island off

West Cork. I had not heard of Sherkin Island but would indeed go to visit if I got the job, so I reassured her. And if I didn't, I'd be back in Ireland soon anyway. So after about half an hour of chatting, Roisin said, "Oh, so you are not looking for midwifery work?" "Well, I said, I'm a bit hard to place as I don't do labour ward and I don't do night duty, so I'm happy to work here in Perth."

"Would you be interested in working in Derby or Fitzroy Crossing?"

Derby, no – I've worked there before, Fitzroy Crossing, yes, but there are no jobs there – my agent has just enquired for me.

Well, I happen to know that there is a vacancy as of today. The midwife who was going from Sydney has pulled out because of the WA lockdown (we had a five day coronavirus lockdown), and her daughter is pregnant, so she doesn't want to risk getting stuck in WA.

"Yes, I'll go to Fitzroy Crossing."

Deepak Chopra calls it synchrodestiny.

I'm sure Roisin nearly fell off her office chair when I said yes. "Do you know where it is?" she asked with a sense of wariness.

"Yes, I drove through it in November. I know the area, so I'm going in with my eyes open."

Then, with whirlwind organisation, I accepted a thirteen-week contract in Fitzroy Crossing as a Community midwife. The following day, I partook in a gruelling Irish interview, sensing clearly that those interviewing me had someone else lined up for the job.

They were seen to be fair.

Fair? Me arse, thinks me.

My philosophical self knows the whole process of application has a purpose. I knew I wanted to go back to London. I would be delighted of course, to be offered the job in Ireland and take it, but I would complete my contract and have a trip to Brisbane to meet up with my Benella midwife colleague Terry and my Tennant Creek teacher friend who both lived close to each other and had started a craft/art business idea together. They were part of my Australian Terracotta Army.

As it happened, I got second place on the panel. This was the second time I had been placed 2nd on the panel. It's an Irish thing. Unlike the first time, I got second when I was the second most successful applicant for midwifery training for a class of twenty. This time it was second on the panel for a job for one.

In other words, I didn't get the job. But then I did. Coronavirus delayed.

Without a blink of regret, I knew I was now planning my return to London. Being in Australia by accident for one year was enough.

I finished my house sit, packed a winter suitcase, including a Trelisa Cooper designer coat I purchased as my prize for getting second place on the Irish panel, and arranged to have it sent off to Highgate. I resent my commissioned aboriginal art that I posted from Tennant Creek last year and which had been returned to Australia via UK customs. Perhaps it will make it to my flat this time? Good old Brexit and customs changes in the UK.

I hoped this would be my last contract in Australia. I started drooling over the road map and planning my route.

Again the car, a Toyota Corolla this time, was all packed and ready for another mammoth journey. I was to start work on March 8th. I'd take four easy days to get there. I might even do some sightseeing on my way.

My brother-in-law is a FIFO worker in the mines. That means he flies in and flies out. He phoned me when he arrived at work the day before I was to leave. "All I could see from the air was flood waters; you might want to check the roads?"

And so I did. Main roads WA has a website that shows all the major roadworks and road closures. That time of year was the tail end of the wet season, and a front had passed by further north. Floods had hit the Great Northern Highway and between Wubin to Paynes, the road was closed. Open to heavy vehicles only.

I was going a different route to that which I had just driven down two months ago. Looking at the road map, I would be driving past

Northam and remembered back to the time when I was working in Australia on one of my contracts in that town.

It is a well-respected secret in a hospital, never to mention the Q word, as once the spell of *quiet* is broken, the guarantee of all hell breaking loose is inevitable.

The small town of Northam, located about three hours from Perth, was not typically busy enough to make the nurses feel overwhelmed during their night shifts. I worked as a midwife there on a short-term contract, Thursday through Sunday. To get to Northam, I would take the train from Perth and be picked up by an orderly at the single-platform station. My accommodation was a dated, dark brown brick flat, which was ideal for sleeping after my shifts. I came fully self-sufficient for meals and did not venture into the town itself, as it had a reputation for being rough.

Memorably for me, Northam was where I learned to play blackjack during the long, mostly uneventful night shifts. Our Enrolled Nurse was, in her former life, a croupier in the casinos of Las Vegas.

I also learned the importance of local knowledge and experience in managing emergencies, especially in a hospital where staffing can be scarce and more is expected of the nursing and midwifery team. The Q word must have slipped passed someone's lips this balmy summer evening because when we arrived for hand over, the place was humming, and people were everywhere. Nothing too serious, but there was no blackjack planned that night. Our team for the night shift at the hospital consisted of Tom, the orderly who, pushing 65, knew everyone in the town and seemed to know what to do and how to do it when it came to the night shift.

Christine, an Enrolled nurse, was a tall and ungainly woman who kept us awake through a shift dealing the cards and telling the tales of her casino days. Milly, an agency staff nurse, was young and pretty with tight ringlets and bleached blonde hair. She was also 26 weeks pregnant and this was her last week at this hospital. Her background was in A&E (Accident and Emergency) and she was an essential complement to me as the midwife. There was a GP who was on call, but as Tom said, he hardly ever saw him come in, preferring to give directions over the phone.

It was about 2am by the time that the few inpatients - all elderly - awaiting rest and home relocation, were settled, and the patients in the ED had all been stitched, cared for and sent home.

All of this had been managed without a doctor on board; such is the running of a rural hospital where it is often hard to get staff and so more is expected of the nursing and midwifery team.

This evening was unusual, as we received a call for a patient experiencing chest pain with an estimated arrival time of seven minutes. The ambulance crew, who were also hospital employees, were on standby at home. Typically, the A&E nurse would take charge of cardiac patients, but Tom, the orderly, stepped up with his calm and experienced voice. Milly and I exchanged glances, with Milly asking how long it had been since I had an MI. I replied that it had been too long, and thanked god for the protocol folder.

In rural hospitals, the protocol folder was the bible of reliability. Easy-to-follow guidelines enabled Millie and me to have the drugs and equipment ready and waiting.

It was clear that Tom was the best person in charge, although upon reflection, it is hard to imagine that ever happening in any city hospital. He directed Christine to prepare the ECG and Defib equipment as well as the observation kit and specimen collections that were tucked away in cupboards I didn't know existed.

He phoned the GP, who was 40 mins away but on her way. It was like a TV sitcom, each of us ready and waiting for the ambulance to arrive.

As Tom opened the large double doors in the ambulance bay, I was shocked to see a slim, middle-aged, well-dressed man, clearly unwell, being rolled in.

Tom was able to find everything we needed. He kept in phone contact with the doctor as Millie and I worked our way methodically through the assessment and initial management process. This man was in trouble. Our eyes communicated the acuity of the situation, and Tom understood.

"We better call the chopper," Tom said. I was surprised to learn that. Realising that the nursing staff could activate the emergency response team without the doctor was something that neither Millie nor I knew. This local knowledge and experience were what I believe saved this man's life.

By the time the GP got to the hospital, the patient had been diagnosed, received first-line drugs, and the helicopter emergency response team had been dispatched from Perth.

As a team, we continued to keep our very unwell gentleman alive. My main job was to push the *shock now* button on the defibrillator. As a midwife and former nurse, this was something I had only done during annual mandatory training. I don't remember how many times the patient went into a shockable rhythm, but each time I called out "All clear! Shock now!" and pressed the button, my stress levels rose along with the patient's as the current passed through his body. The patient remained conscious, but his eyes appeared dark.

Where the hell was the rescue team?

I secretly wondered how many more defibrillations this man could tolerate. My colleagues too looked very worried. Then Tom got the call. ETA nine minutes.

I think that was the longest nine minutes of my nursing career. Mags, the very butch and personable GP, was talking with the cardiology team in Perth; Milly was administering drugs, noting observations, and documenting our care.

Tom had gone outside to meet the chopper crew at the helipad.

Our patient was stable on the resus trolley. The ECG monitor was beeping away. The three of us were all deep in our own thoughts when through the curtains, came the form of our Medic. Dressed in red overalls with Doctor Tim on his left breast pocket, this tall slim, and deliciously good-looking dark-haired man said, "Hi team, how's it going here? Looking good," he said in a deep and confident tone as he glanced first at the patient, then the ECG monitor, and back over the IV fluids.

For the briefest of moments, Pregnant Millie, Butch GP Mags, and Married Midwife Me shared a look acknowledging the handsomeness of our rescuer before delving into the handover.

With time bound efficiency, our patient was transferred to the Medical Team and soon we were left with the rush of cool air and the noisy thudding as the helicopter disappeared into the night.

We three stood there watching the chopper lights fade away. Relief and tiredness hit us as we all burst into laughter – each knowing it was about the god-like rescuer that had emerged through the bedside curtains.

Tom looked at us as though we were all crazy.

I don't think he would have understood.

That was a dreamy memory of the sleepy wee town.

More of a nightmare memory was another night shift when a young indigenous woman arrived from her community to the ward about 11pm. When she walked in I saw a heavily pregnant woman, an older grey haired woman at her side followed by two younger girls who were laughing and messing. The other woman who looked unkempt was her mother.

Relieved that Carina had arrived, my assessment started. She was holding her pregnant bellie and was walking easily. "I think the baby is coming," said the older woman who was a grandmother.

We went into the birthing room and the support women came in as is quite usual.

My colleague got Milo and biscuits for them.

I asked Carina what was happening and did she think the baby was coming? She didn't seem to be in labour to me. Grandmother said, "She got a pain in her guts sister, been there all day I think the baby's coming."

Carina had not said anything and as she got onto the examination couch I could see she was obviously in pain.

The other three women had left and were outside in a waiting area. I asked Carina to show me where the pains were. "Here" she said circling the whole of her abdomen, "been sore all day."

I felt the tension of her stomach and the words of my Limerick Maternity Tutor hit me. "rock hard abdomen = placental abruption".

This was an obstetric emergency. I phoned the GP who was relieved I was there as he said he knew nothing about obstetrics and agreed to proceed to emergency transfer to King Edward Hospital in Perth.

The system was in place and without delay Carina and I were in the back of the ambulance with a trainee ambulance volunteer who insisted on taking systolic blood pressure and doing a pain score. There were two drivers upfront.

It was the first (and only) time I had felt some disconnect with the ambulance staff. I couldn't put my finger on what was happening but in the end, I was asking why we were driving at normal speed not with the lights and sirens towards Perth.

"You didn't ask for it to be blue lighted" said the woman driver. The man sitting next to her looked straight ahead.

"I didn't know I had to – I told you it was an obstetric emergency. I thought that would be enough?"

"Oh you are from New Zealand aren't you? No you don't know the important stuff do you?"

I was stumped. "This is an obstetric emergency, please drive with blue lights" I said with a dollop of sarcasm internally fuming at her belligerent anti- Kiwi racism. The lights went on and the we speeded up.

The team at Perth were at the ambulance bay to meet us and as it happened they knew me, so trusted my diagnosis. Carina went directly for c/section and both mum and bub were healthy.

With such relief at having got Carina to the hospital, I reflected on how amazing the indigenous women are. They knew when to get help and drove all those hours with women supporting women. My contribution was a minor part.

I was mentally exhausted on the return journey. The ambulance called into a servo to refuel and for the crew to get something to eat.

I had left my wallet at Northam. Unbelievably the power and control freak of an ambulance driver, instead of buying me a coffee as most colleagues would, just said, "Well, you won't forget next time, will you?"

Her fellow driver waited for her to be out of earshot. "Do you want me to lend you some money?"

Fighting back the tears, I declined.

32 ON THE ROAD AGAIN: PERTH TO FITZROY CROSSING

This trip was stymied. The bureau of meteorology (BOM) forecast more rain, and that would mean more flooding.

I called my accommodation at the Cue hotel, where I had booked a room for the first night, to let them know about the road closure. The lady I spoke with was understanding and reassured me that the flood waters often receded quickly. She said she would wait until the next day to cancel my reservation, and advised me to call back at lunchtime if the road was still closed.

As it turned out, the flood waters did recede by 8:37am the next day, and the main roads were updated to allow for light vehicles to proceed with caution. I ended up leaving a couple of hours later than planned, but I was confident that I would arrive before sunset. In the past, I had driven past many floodways and wondered what they would be like during wet weather, but I had never experienced it firsthand. I knew that my small Toyota Corolla wouldn't be able to handle driving through any water on the road, so I was careful to avoid it. My BB (big brother) had also explained the physics of how flowing water can be dangerous for small vehicles, so I was already wary of the risk.

He suggested I walk it to check, if I was worried.

I located my walking pole, made sure my sandals were handy on the back seat and set off to Cue via the previously flooded roads.

Anxiously anticipating some surprise flood waters around Wagin, all that was left was red dirt and branch debris that had been washed across the highway. The fields had pockets of water. The trees in places took on a stranded island look, their trunks surrounded by red water. On the sides of one of the floodways, the flow was fast, and it was sobering to see the volume and velocity of a raging stream when the sky was clear blue.

On other trips, I had noticed the angled paths branching off from the main roads and wondered what they were for. These single lane paths, with chevron-like markings, can be found throughout Australia. I had previously thought they were where dirt was deposited when the roads were constructed, but I now understand that they are part of a flood control system. These paths divert floodwaters and channel rainwater that falls on distant lands, nourishing the desert as it passes by.

Today spring green pockets of new growth splatter amongst the red. A hint of mauve is about to bud and celebrate the rainfall.

The long-awaited rains are to come.

The long-awaited rains go.

***

Cue was a curiosity and convenient stop-off point. About fifty kilometres to the destination, I found myself pulling in behind an escort vehicle with flashing lights. Further ahead, I could see the large mechanical form spanning both lanes of the highway.

People often ask if I get bored when I'm driving so far. So much fascinates me in the simple changes of landscapes from flat to flatter, trees to dirt, crazy-shaped rocks to mining hills covered in moss. I don't think that I've actually been bored. I've been bored with my audiobook. I've been bored with podcasts. But not bored with the drive.

The sight ahead of me caught my attention. There were what appeared to be two separate vehicles. The one at the front was box-shaped, as wide as both lanes, and towering in height. The second was lower and narrower, but two lateral pieces were protruding to equal the width of the former. Neither were identifiable to me. They were the biggest pieces of kit I had ever seen travelling on the road. It was incredible. There is always a lot of talk about how big the machinery and operations in the mines are, but as I had never been to a site, I didn't appreciate the truth in this tale. Following behind this monstrosity was fascinating.

Three road trains caught up with the slowed traffic.

In my wee Toyota Corolla, I was like an ant amongst giants. I had nowhere to go but to follow the white van with its flashing lights. The convoy travelled at 30kph for 30 minutes, then was diverted through a roadside parking bay with slick logistics, and within ten minutes, I had arrived at my destination.

I took a few sneaky photos while driving behind the convoy and discovered the machinery to be that of a Liebherr mining excavator. About two hours after checking into my hotel, I was sitting on the upstairs verandah when the convoy drove past. This time I could see the size and form in greater detail. The first set had a front truck attached to a second truck, towing the large square kit. I think the two motors gave more towing power. The following machine was attached to the single cab. The convoy was led by two for vehicles, and wondered about the incredible piece of machinery. I doubt I will ever see such a sight again.

Or so I thought.

My excitement was not quite the same the next morning when I met up with them! I'd had enough wonderment. Luckily, I got waved through relatively quickly. Somehow I wouldn't be surprised if we met on the road again.

The Queen of the Murchison, Cue was the only available accommodation. Ruth had reassured me and did not cancel my booking, so when I arrived, she spoke to me like an old friend. The accommodation and café were in the centre of the town of Cue. The main street boasted grand buildings with ornate verandas that I had now come to expect in rural Australia. Sadly, this town has seen better days. The infamous Queen of the Murchison was a rabbit warren of rooms in various states of either packing up to close or storing for renovations. Ruth took me to my allocated room up a sweeping deep wooded stairway. "The bannister was newly oiled," she said, "that's why it's a bit tacky to touch."

I looked warily at the wood. It did look tacky – was I relieved to know it wasn't grime? Maybe a little.

The key to my room had gone missing, but Ruth said she would try to find it. I was shown my king-single room, nicely presented with a shaving kit, slippers, and a dressing gown. Then the grand tour led me past a young man hammering down new vinyl flooring that was being replaced, because Ruth's husband had got a dog which had upset the cat, who pissed in the hallway.

Along two corridors, I was shown the ladies' facilities. Oh shit! A rooky mistake of mine not to notice the lack of ensuite. But I could tell this was accommodation for the miners, so I would probably have the bathroom to myself.

Now the dressing gown made sense.

Down another flight of stairs to a dining room with a continental breakfast facility, where I could help myself to tea and coffee. My car could be parked out the back, past the un-manned Caltex, along the fence line and into the first gate. Ruth would just use the card I booked with, and did I still want dinner, or would I go across the road to the pub?

I was speechless. My children had booked me a luxury hotel stay in Perth for my birthday the weekend prior. I hadn't mentally adjusted to manage my expectations and needed a moment to remember that I was again in the rural Australian mining district.

It would be ok.

"I'll go across the road to the pub," I said, "Thank you." Cat piss and sticky balustrades were still at the forefront of my mind.

Ruth didn't find the Room 2 key. I didn't think I needed it anyway. After pub grub across the road at the *'far cue bar,'* I returned to the Queen of the Murchison. The first-floor veranda swept wide around the building. The holes in her floorboards had potted plants to cover the evidence of disrepair and age. I sipped my tea and looked up to the night sky, where the southern cross again caressed me with her aroha.

Back in my room, I left the curtains undrawn, hoping the view of the stars would woo me to sleep.

A canister of Raid on the bedside cabinet hinted they wouldn't.

The drive to Newman was as uneventful as is the town. Curiosity ignited my desire to go to a mine site but it was met with disappointment as the infamous mine tour was no longer happening due to coronavirus.

My midwifery buddy phoned me to check in on me. In the way that random events happen, Michelle reminded me that she had been to Newman on an ill-fated trip with her now ex-husband as his appendix was threatening to burst. We both took a moment at that memory. It was me who had said, "Pity it hadn't?" as we laughed at the black humour. The ex husband had gone on to win the WA lottery that gave him a couple of million dollars and a house in Hillarys Harbour, Perth's prestigious real estate. Last my friend had heard, he was living on a Coral Island as a caretaker off the coast of Queensland. Yip.

***

Next stop, Port Headland.

I hadn't stopped in Port Headland on my drive south at the end of 2020. At that time I had actually been disconcerted as it was the first time I had driven through a sand storm. The roads newly sealed were grey and the markings startlingly white. In contrast, the sky took on a dark ominous look as the wind whipped up the red sands blowing them high enough to colour the white clouds. Small patches of blue would appear amidst dirty dust. I didn't know if I should stop and let the storm pass, or continue. A few other vehicles continued through the storm so I decided to box on through to Karratha. It was one of the few times my confidence in my journey was rattled.

This time I had travelled the inland route, and Port Hedland was where I would need to stay. I haven't changed my opinion of the industrial settlement, and although there are always midwifery jobs going, I didn't feel the need to work there. My overnight stay was easy, and I learned that flatback turtles nest there, but I didn't see any. Just the wrong time of year.

I had only ever seen one turtle and that was in Sardinia. They usually live to an old age, unless someone stands on them, which I had. In fairness, the Air BNB had promised a surprise in their garden. I was not expecting to see their pet turtle as I hung out my washing.

I was starting to think ahead to the women and my role in Fitzroy Crossing with renewed enthusiasm. I really did like community midwifery outback style and hoped it would be a good contract.

33 BACK TO WORK

It seemed a little surreal. The accommodation I was booked into for my orientation was an upmarket complex, with a pool, restaurant, and bar. My conscience pricked for a tiny minute, wondering why the health budget would pay for this, but I quickly got over it. For now, I would relax and enjoy the decadence, soak up all the training, and mentally prepare for life in Fitzroy crossing.

I ordered a glass of Prosecco and sat beside the pool.

Cheers, Slānte, *Kia ora*.

I could just about manage this until I got back to London and was starting to look forward to the challenge.

In my orientation, I was bombarded with Acronyms. I know Ozzie health is full of them, but they went overboard in the community health service. Those in the know, spoke this new acronym language. I just stayed quiet, figuring I would eventually pick up what was what. In all honesty, I don't think I actually did. It took me a while to realise that I was being employed by a very different organisation than I had worked under previously. Western Australia Community Health Service (WACHS) has its own way, its own budget, and that is all I'm going to say about that.

I took myself off to one of the local haunts after work.

And I wrote a piece for my creative writing homework. Our group were still meeting via zoom on Wednesday's.

Birds are squawking and fussing in competition to the upbeat playlist coming from the speakers discreetly placed amongst the outdoor seating. The noisy critters are settling in for the night amongst the palm tree tops that are rustling in the gentle breeze, the trunks erect yet on a permanent lean. These happy trees bend and bow to the cyclone when it hits.

It's early in the evening. The sun is yet to set. That's what the attraction is. The trestle tables and bar stools have a scattering of patrons, men with beer wrapped in the stubby holder, women who sip from delicate shaped glasses. Before long, the workers will arrive to celebrate the end of the day and the tourists will ply themselves with Deet to deter the mosquitos that prefer some hot blood to cocktails. Frangipani scent lingers at the entrance. Chemical warfare is needed inside.

Most patrons have their shades on and are looking out beyond the mangroves and bushes that carpet the seafront directly in front of this swanky hotel garden. One lonely rock is the only interruption along the calm blue sea from coast to horizon. There is something visible far away but indiscernible, perhaps an oil platform, or an atoll or landmass that the navigators will know about. For now, I sit and sip my priscroppino cocktail recommended by the Spanish waitress and constructed with knowledge by the hands of the French barista. But for the heat hanging, I could forget where I am. It is always best to make the days count rather than count the days.

My two days of orientation to prepare me for working for WACHS completed; New passwords, new IT systems, new paperwork, new policies, new acronyms new management structure. It is the most tiresome part of being a mobile midwife - every contract is always new.

I waved goodbye to my decadent resort hotel accommodation and drove to Fitzroy Crossing.

FROM CITY LIGHTS TO OUTBACK NIGHTS   183

It was the weirdest De ja vous.

34 FIRES, PLAGUE, THEN FLOODS.

The wet season in the Kimberley region of Western Australia is from November through to April. The rain falls in short heavy downpours, often accompanied by electrical storms. Dramatic sunsets are a photographer's delight. This is not the time for tourists as the humidity, and sticky heat is burdensome. The pesky flies love the wet season, and the mosquitos are the size of a single-engine Cessna.

I arrived at my new placement towards the end of the wet season. Word on the street was that it had been a 'good wet', meaning there had been sufficient rain to ward off drought, and we were not to expect much more rain.

But rain it did.

The big wet started on a Tuesday. First, there were the puddles. The bush telegraph warned that the BP station, where the sandwiches are made fresh every day, had too much surface flooding for the smaller vehicles to drive through.

Then the dirt roads started to get deep rivets making the driving with the 4X4 difficult but a truck load of fun to negotiate. Then the floodways' were covered with surface water, and by the Thursday morning, these had become invisible. The indigenous were swimming, enjoying the cool fresh, clean water. By late Thursday afternoon, the channel that had a one-way bridge crossing had burst its banks. The lands out to the main highway had turned into picturesque tree lakes, each specimen mirrored in the still fresh water as if Swan Lake was being reimagined for the Kimberly wet.

It was the mighty Fitzroy river that caused most conversation and speculation.

The river reports posted on the local social media sites would be in stiff competition to the BBC4 shipping forecast.

Fitzroy River Level @Fitzroy Crossing 10.947m and STEADY @3pm
Fitzroy river Level @ Dimond Gorge 7.068m and RISING @3pm
Margaret River @Margaret Gorge 1.0707m and RISING @3pm.

The excitement was palpable.

'It hadn't been this wet since?' Well, that had various answers, and the debate continued. It was coming to the end of the week, and the roads out of Fitzroy Crossing had closed.

We were stuck. The indigenous were stuck. From the air, the communities were now small islands.

Islands in the desert.

The key to personal survival in Fitzroy Crossing is to learn the local knowledge. Revered seemingly as much as the London cabbies' knowledge, this remote community thrives on teaching its newcomers the most important key points of information.

On my first day, as part of my orientation, I was taken on a tiki tour of the town. I can call it a tiki tour because Ata is a Maori woman from the north island, and we have Whānau, family connections. Roads and communities were pointed out. Who lived where, what road led to the art centre, and how to find my way to the IGA. It seemed I was driven in a never ending loop, so by the end of my tiki tour, I had no fecking idea where I was. Then I recognised the servo from my first stop to fill my tank with petrol the day I had arrived.

With all seriousness, Ata announced. "This is where you get

coffee - 2 dollars and 50 cents for a large one. But don't buy sandwiches here. They are frozen Coles brand, and they are always stale."

Friday is an admin day in community health, but the flights and road trips to the communities had been disrupted all week. There was a sense of frustration and urgency. There had been no medicines to the communities, and no nurse visits for over a week. A helicopter was booked to take two nurses, a doctor, and prescriptions, but the low visibility accompanying the rain put the proverbial dampener on that plan.

The office was abuzz with who was stuck where, who was trying to get where and with a palpable resignation to the helplessness lay a blanket of disquiet.

Then pizzas arrived.

Management in Broome had ordered fresh from the local resorts' oven, a treat to cheer everyone on. It worked, except for the office humbug who totted up the bill and curiously noted what the money could have been better spent on. (like what? paper clips or syringes?)

News kept coming in from the local Aboriginal Liaison Officers (ALOs) of the road closures, locals getting stuck, and cars getting caught in rising waters. There was an excitement underpinning the gossip.

Rules and Regulations that would govern a city hospital have little place in rural Australia when natural disasters hit. At the beginning of the flood closures, one of the remote communities had an emergency. The low clouds prohibited any air rescue, so the ambulance team retrieved a decommissioned vehicle they knew would have a good shot at managing the flood waters, cranked her up, and headed along the 80km drive. Sadly, the patient passed away and would not have had any better outcome had the team gotten there earlier. But knowing that all was being done, I hope, was some consolation.

Later in the week, Alistair, a Kiwi helicopter pilot who escaped Nepal at the beginning of the pandemic and was now also a coronavirus refugee in Oz, was brought in to deliver medications to the island communities. The logistics necessitated a Registered nurse to accompany the delivery, the male ALO Jason, for cultural liaison, and a Registered nurse to receive. A few hands went up for this job. Such wonderful opportunities we can be presented with when working remote. After the drug run, we all oggled over the photos. The ALO gave us geographical landmarks of the river ways snaking through the land and her spills reaching out indiscriminately, claiming the soils. Roads weaved in and out of view as they were flooded. Jason showed us where the locals would, in a couple of days, drive to and take a boat to meet a vehicle on the other side. True to the tale, some of the Noonkanbah community slowly made it into the town. Pop up casinos and drinking circles formed. The hospital was eerily quiet.

Many long-termers said the amount of rain this season is above and beyond most memory. Despite the inconvenience, the wet was welcomed.

Small groups of locals gathered with their 'tinnies' to sit and yarn down the creek. The younger ones were swimming impervious to the water snakes and freshwater crocodiles I would have been worried about. It took me back to my days in Derby when I first experienced the rain in the wet. I was at Woollies doing a shop when seemingly out of nowhere, the heavens opened, and the locals emerged to stand and soak up the cooling water in the middle of the car park. Unlike Gene Kelly in the cold dark streets of NY, in Derby the light was tempered by the transient clouds that were billowy white, the temperature steamy hot, and the clear, warm drops of rain falling on the dark aboriginal skin of dancing people oozed simple joy.

Back on the Fitzroy River, the older kids were jumping off the bridge into the fast-flowing river. Terrifying to watch. But the freedom and delight was palpable.

The FX hospital and Community health service share a work site, but there is a demarcation line that both Kiwis and short-term contractors can't figure out. At the main entrance, a security guard vets who is allowed in and who is not. This includes if anyone has been drinking or appears to be humbugging. Suppose you make it through to the foyer. In that case, there is a reception desk; however, if you want the community health services for maternity, sexual health, or general enquiries, you are almost always ignored and eventually directed through the door, which is locked, so you need to ring the bell and hope that Ata or someone is actually in their office to answer the door. It is neither client friendly nor culture-centric. Mostly, the pregnant women just hang about the side door until the midwife looks for them and finds them waiting. At the back of this hospital wing is an Indigenous-funded service. They have meeting spaces outside under the trees, a kitchen, and food available. Most of the signs and information show some attempt to be of interest for them to decipher. There are fewer words, more pictures, and indigenous faces.

Off the other wing is the hospital with outpatient offices, teaching rooms, and in patient wards. This is also where the Emergency department is housed. This seems to be oversubscribed with seriously unwell or road traffic crash victims.

Both the community health and the hospital, although under the same roof, have completely different funding, supply, staff, medications, policies, and procedures.

I found this frustrating and obstructive to providing care to the community. I felt that it would serve the people better if a more cooperative approach functioned. When a pregnant woman needed an iron infusion which was becoming a more and more popular means of treating iron deficiency in pregnancy, as a midwife employed by Community Health, I could not administer IV drugs. The client would need to be admitted as a day stay or short stay admission to the ED, the community health doctor if one was actually happy to do so would need to prescribe the medication. Alternatively, I would have to contact the registrar or locum obstetric doctor in Derby a town which was three hours drive away. They would then need to fax the prescription and follow through by posting through internal mail the original prescription. Then the midwife would need to have the laboratory results, the prescription, and the dispensed medication prepared and ready. An appointment would then be made in the double staff time and the nursing staff from the ED would administer the iron infusion.

This whole process had so many junctions of failure that the efforts often failed. The challenge of getting the mums from their communities into a hospital at a specific time of day and returning them back to their homes was impossible. I started to become frustrated.

Get Rocked.

Alice Springs was on the news last night. Out-of-control kids throwing rocks as soon as the sun sets. The town is in a state of anarchy.

I had heard of this happening when I lived there, but the trend has also hit FX (Fitzroy Crossing). Over two evenings, I was a target of getting rocked. I don't take it personally.

Like Forrest Gump's box of chocolates, the accommodation provided with the jobs in rural Australia was inconsistent. The house I was allocated in FX had boarded-up windows and overgrown grass. Located on the corner of a road with field access to the local servo and a well-trodden pathway, it felt exposed.

One interesting concept that I've noticed all over the outback towns is the concept of normalisation. When I was taken to the house, Ata, who was not only the Community Health Administrative Assistant but also a self-appointed accommodation officer, said, "Oh, you will love this house. Look at the big kitchen. Oh a dishwasher! Look at the big bedrooms."

We wandered through the 3-bedroom purpose-built house owned by a local Aboriginal corporation and leased to the health board for a breath-taking weekly amount. I was unimpressed. It felt dodgy. It was referred to as the big brother house amongst the staff.

"Why are the windows here and upstairs boarded over?" I asked. "Oh, that's for your safety." "When I lived here," said Ata, "we had a home invasion." She went on to describe what had happened, how the police were on a job in a community out of town, and how the "little shits" kept on trashing the place while still inside. She then said she had a friend there also, so she didn't feel so scared.

"The windows are boarded up, so if they smash it, they can't get their arm around the corner to open the door," she continued.

I was not impressed. I said I didn't like it. I was told that because I didn't want to share it's the best they could do. Other houses were too expensive to open. I thought it was just what I had to accept.

Once I moved in, I noticed the safety alarm didn't work, the lights were blown in a couple of rooms, and the large ranch slider window sat precariously in its frame.

Then I got rocked.

A colleague was having a cuppa with me when it first happened. It gave me a start. Unsure of how to react, I instinctively wanted to call the police. But Wendy has a calm manner and went out to meet the aggressors. I slunk sheepishly behind her. I thought, maybe this is just normal here? I'd better not make a fuss.

Standing at the gate was a group of eight or nine-year-old boys, who apparently were not the ones who were throwing the rocks, but they were more than happy to dob in their buddy. "And he did that too, Miss," pointing to the graffiti inside the green big brother style fence. "Miss, Miss, it wasn't us Miss, it was Troy from that house."

Five young boys were all pointing to the house two or maybe three doors along. I didn't need to know.

Wendy had dissipated my angst, and I was impressed with her manner.

It was her second tour of Fitzroy. She seemed to be unperturbed by this behaviour. Two days later, when round two happened, I was less calm. This time their aim and persistence ended with my bathroom window smashed in.

The town was flooded, there was no transport in or out, and I was not going to stay and get rocks thrown through my windows.

I had no way of escape. It is an incredibly foreign feeling to be physically isolated and marooned, but I was determined to remain calm.

I was not, however, going to accept this as a normal way of living.

I was clear with my concerns and expectations. I felt that somehow I was being set up by being housed there. My suspicion was confirmed a few weeks down the track. Ata had some strange ways.

Incensed, I phoned my managers in Broome, who immediately arranged for me to stay in the local lodge until I could move into a share house after the weekend.

On the quiet, I had forewarned Wendy what had happened and that Ata insisted that I move into the shared accommodation with her. We had agreed on this idea as we already formed a rapport. However, Wendy's fairly new man friend was coming through FX for work, and they had planned a bit of a romantic weekend. I did not want to play gooseberry. When Ata called, Wendy didn't answer her phone.

As it happened, her friend got stranded by the weather. I stayed in the lodge and moved in on Monday. The next week, Wendy also had another meeting with a different gang of tender-aged vagabonds. This time a small child's hand was presented "Look what I've got," he announced. "A lighter?" said Calm Wendy, just as he launched at her with a knife edge, as though to slice her arm, demanding her money. Calm Wendy acted perplexed and said, 'Im out for a walk, I don't have any money. The boys ran away.

I fear for Fitzroy Crossing.

I moved into a shared house with Wendy and I shared the house and became great friends. I thoroughly enjoyed her company and that of the other three households of nurses in the same small complex.

People and Places

It is said that the Fitzroy River has the propensity to fill the Sydney harbour many times over when it floods. The exact number of times changes from storyteller to storyteller, but watching her girth expand with increasing velocity measured against the bridge stays, is evidence that this is a movable beast. The volume of water flowing this season was consuming the locals with wonder. Bob , a helicopter engineer who has lived in the crossing for many moons, got his boat out, filled the jerry cans with diesel, and took a few of us upriver to Danggu, formerly known as Geikie Gorge. "Hold on to your hat," he hollered as we powered along a flooded tar-sealed Ytani road, slipped under a tree-lined former riverbank, and out into the swiftly flowing waters heading upstream. It is almost unfathomable that we were now in a boat, where one week earlier we had driven. Half an hour into our trip, we passed the Brooking Channel and Margaret River branches feeding the Fitzroy. These are popular walking spots in the dry. Beyond, the low-lying land and grass-covered banks expand into an eye-wateringly beautiful gorge.

Danggu.

This gorge has been carved out by the Fitzroy River through limestone that was originally a reef. Bob , now turned tour guide, explained it as *being formed by organisms that shit limestone, and it sounds weird but is apparently true.*

Impressively, algae and lime excreting organisms have worked away doing what they do best to form this mass of two kilometre high rocks. I didn't see any fossils; however, it is known they are there if you know what to look for. What I saw were magnificent slate brown-red rocks shaped by rain and wind into statues and monuments to nature over the thousands of years, rogue trees and an occasional brilliant green tiny plant that has happened to grow on an opportunistic ledge.

We pulled in alongside a deep tunnelling hole in the rock that was cascading fresh, deliciously soft water, which we all drank. This hole in the rock is inaccessible by ordinary means. Today mother nature shared her spoils.

Downstream we were battered more by the current; Bob skilfully avoiding rogue trees and debris. Making a speedy right turn, we coasted into the parking area for the Danggu boat tour ramps, where in the dry season, many tourists are whisked away into the gorge or walk along the mostly dry riverbeds.

What a marvel awaited us. I had been to this parking area, read the information on the gazebo and walked down to the river to look at the gorge. Now I was in a boat being driven around the car park, the signs only peeping above the water line. The water level was at the roof of the information kiosk. My boat colleague stepped onto the roof for a rare photo opportunity.

A week after the floods, the car park was covered in silt, the only evidence of flooding.

I'm one of the lucky people who have had this exposure to the wilds of the outback.

Bob had taken a trip earlier in the morning and had managed to go under the main highway bridge. Three hours later, the water had risen, so we could not risk decapitation.

We made our way back to the road where we were launched from, again negotiating the water on the road to be greeted by a police utility vehicle.

Two uniformed officers were leaning on their open doors like a couple of cowboys watching the boat navigate along the former road. The banter began about who they were waiting for. Bob steered the boat up and we hopped out into the water and up onto the dry. The police officers were checking out who was breaking the law and driving along the closed roads. The older of the two said 'who am I to stand in the way of such good fun?'

I'm pretty sure Bob had another river run at the end of their shift.

35 COVID STONE AND COVID GREY

It's been a year now since the first coronavirus case in Australia.

My Whānau in NZ, London, Latvia, Belgium, France, Spain, and Australia have two things in common.

It's called the Covid stone and Covid grey.

If you are not sure what it means, it is that most will have put on weight and been deprived of access to hairdressers.

No one predicted this trend.

I'm already in one camp, and the lack of a hair salon within 500 kilometres means I will need to dip my toe in the other.

Braving the Dogs

During my stay in Australia through the pandemic, I've failed to keep fit. In spite of time, beautiful weather, and not much else to do. The incessant heat, flies, mosquitos, and my fear of dogs was spiralling me into inactivity. In the Northern Territory, camp dogs have been renamed *cheeky dogs, which* evokes sympathy and compassion.

Fitzroy Dogs are still camp dogs. The previous November, when I had passed through and done a reiki session for my friend, I had seen no stray animals and had been lulled into thinking the vet neutering scheme initiated when Michelle had lived here many years ago, had worked.

I was mistaken. The dogs spotted me on my first day in residence. The mongrel mix were breeds that, in my mind, were the vicious Pitbull, Staffie, and Alsatian, ready to bite me, or worse, chase me. Even if they were behind their owner's fence, the aggressive barking was enough to send my flight or fight response into overdrive. The thought of going for a walk was seemingly impossible.

My coronavirus stone was ever-present. I missed walking. I would be brave and get out.

On the first Sunday in my share flat, I woke early and made the decision to take the advice of my colleagues: walk early to avoid the heat, mozzies', and pesky out-of-control kids. Go out of the main town towards the airport where there are no camp dogs, never look any dog in the eye, walk assertively, and if you really want to, take a walking pole.

I woke up at 5:30 in the morning when the natural light streamed into my room. Deciding to take advantage of the early hour, I put on my walking shoes and made my way outside, trying to ignore the anxiety that had been bothering me. As I walked through the streets of Fitzroy, I noticed something I hadn't before - a quiet and peaceful stillness that only a few early birds seemed to share. The warm air was refreshing as I stepped up my pace, feeling a sense of relief wash over me as I pushed past my worries and fears. It was a small victory, but an important one nonetheless.

As I approached the footbridge, I couldn't help but notice the aftermath of the recent flood. Straggly pieces of bush, branches, and silty mud were caught in the wires, evidence of the water that had once rushed through the area. Though the creek still had some remnants of water left, it too would soon disappear. And then, as if waiting for me, a dog appeared out of nowhere. My instincts in - my dog radar had detected a camp dog, triggering my sympathetic nervous system and a rush of adrenaline. But then, I remembered the advice I had been given: don't make eye contact and walk assertively. I wished I had my walking pole with me but continued towards the bridge. The dog remained still, watching my every move. My heart was pounding - should I acknowledge the dog or ignore it? I quickened my pace, my steps in sync with my racing heart. Out of the corner of my eye, the supposed vicious camp dog remained still, his tongue hanging freely and wagging his tail - he seemed harmless to me.

Aaah, nice doggie, I said intuitively, and his tail wagged a little more. I relaxed, maybe camp dogs are not so bad after all.

I clomped across the bridge, and the dog followed me, totally unperturbed by the wire footing, which I would have thought his little paw might fall through. A work colleague lived on the other side of this bridge, and there was a town camp beyond, so I thought the dog was going home.

He happily walked just at my heel as if I had spent time and effort at dog training camp. Knowing he would soon stop or continue ahead to his home, I took a left turn up the road towards the main road and airport.

The dog followed.

"Go home," I said. He didn't understand me. "Home! Shoo, away you go," I barked at him. He stopped and looked me in the eye and wagged his tail. I carried on walking. A car was coming from the main road, so I stepped off into the grass side strip. The dog stayed on the road, and the car was coming straight towards him. I became his protector waving my arms and yelling at him to shoo him off the road. The dog stayed still. The car stopped.

It was now 6 am, and the car with windows down, had a driver and three passengers.

"Is this your dog?" I asked. "No that's Prince," said the young fellow behind the driver, who took a gulp from his emu can. "Do you want him?" he asked.

" No, I don't want a dog. He's following me – can you take him home?" I asked.

"We'll pickhimuponthewayback," said the driver.

"Donworryhe'llbealrighthe'llfindhiswayhome.

You from New Zealand?" the other young man in the back asked.

"Yes, I am," I said instinctively, putting my hand to the pounamu I always wear.

"Yeahiknowaboutthosethings - that green stone keeps you safe miss," he said.

"Seeyamiss," said the driver, and they drove towards dog, now known as Prince, who casually walked out of their way.

The lads carried on the road, and I saw the spray of floodwater that still covered the causeway. They would have been soaked. They would be all laughing at that, I imagined.

The car did another floodwater drive-through and, as they passed, didn't pick up Prince but drove on by. Unbelievable, I thought.

Prince faithfully accompanied me past the airport along the hospital road and back to my house. By this time, I found myself talking to him, but he still didn't seem to know what I was saying. Back at the flat, I went inside to get the car keys. Prince didn't ask to come inside; I think he knew he would be pushing his luck. I opened the car, and he happily hopped in. If only my friends could see me now, I thought to myself and smiled. Prince stood on the back seat, his front paws on the passenger's headrest, his little white face next to mine.

I told him my plan. He didn't reply, so I assumed he was happy with that. At the IGA, I wound the window down a bit to let air flow through. It was my lucky day. Dog food was on special. I purchased a $1.75 can of beef and vegetables.

When I arrived back at the car, Prince was not there.

The bloody dog had jumped out the window, and I thought he had wandered off. But around the other side of the car, there he was, standing as if he had been at the bridge all the time, waiting for me.

He jumped back into the vehicle, and we drove back to the footbridge where we had met.

He seemed happy with the plan when the delicious meat, disguised as beef, was served on the flattish rock next to the bridge. I drove away, hoping like hell Prince wouldn't be one of those car-chasing dogs.

But of course, he wasn't.

He didn't even say thank you.

36 A DAY IN THE LIFE OF A MIDWIFE - FITZROY STYLE

It is true for any midwife that no day will ever be the same. You never know what will come through the door in a box of chocolate Forrest Gump kind of way.

Fitzroy is considered a remote community. The problems with alcohol induced violence, both domestic and community, has caused the powers that be, AKA Federal Government, to categorise it as a dry community. This means that grog can be purchased with a meal, and people can drink in their own home, but there is no Bottle-O. The closest outlet is Derby, 250 Km. Or Broome 400km away, a similar distance as London to Glasgow. The closest mainstream supermarket is Derby, so if you were to make a comparison, it would get you from London to Manchester.

There is a library in the town, an IGA supermarket, two petrol stations that sell hot food, two hotels, one camping ground, and a footy oval.

And, of course, a hospital.

It was my third week, and I was getting to meet some of the pregnant women under my care.

We had three women in need of sit-down appointments or pregnancy management services, and Broome or Derby were the closest locations for these services. Sit down is the pre-arranged time about 2-4 weeks before the baby is due to be born. However, getting there was proving to be a challenge due to the recent flood. The roads were still closed, making travel by car impossible. The only option was to fly, but the Fitzroy airport was bustling with activity - it seemed like every service in and out of town was using it. Hospital flights were taking priority, understandably, but it was making it difficult for our women to secure a flight. We knew we had to find a solution soon, as these appointments were crucial for the health of the women and their babies.

Adelina was having her first baby. She had been diagnosed with RHD rheumatic heart disease when she was nine and had had surgery at the age of thirteen; now she was eighteen, pregnant, and needed close monitoring of her cardiac function. Health is not always a priority for our indigenous people. Appointments are made and ignored. Transport and accommodation are booked for each outpatient visit, and it is more likely that any one person will have two or three scheduled times to see a specialist before they actually attend.

This is frustrating and time-consuming. We document it. Our vocabulary and documentation must be as non-judgmental as a simple 'did not attend' (DNA). We might be tempted, but we can't accuse the women of being non-compliant. Most of us accept this and keep trying to motivate and encourage them to *comply*, giving all the health benefits to entice them. Patient assisted travel service (PATS) clerical workers seem intolerant and belligerent behind their bureaucratic desks. It was as though the money was coming out of their pay check, not the government funds.

Through my experience working with indigenous clients, I have come to learn that they have a unique sense of timing. While their arrival at appointments may be preceded by a flurry of urgent phone calls, texts and demands, they always seem to show up at the right time on the right day. It can be nerve-wracking waiting for their confirmation, but once we receive it, we're relieved that they're going to make the appointment. We keep answering their calls until the very last moment, when chocks away is called, or the pilot starts attending to the plane. It's only when we see a little face through the Perspex window of the tiny plane that we can mentally tick the box of completion. It's always a pleasant surprise, and we've come to appreciate their unique sense of timing.

On my second trip to the airport for the day, I waved Adelina off. Her little face looking out of the window showed angst. She told me that being on a plane is pretty scary, but ok. She had flown before, but not alone.

I now have to hope like hell that the Broome end of the journey can be completed and that Adelina gets to the echocardiograph appointment. Then, more importantly, we learn her fragile heart has responded to the syrupy injection of Bicillin that we inject into the butt muscle every month.

Natalia is expecting her second baby. She is twenty one and is due in three weeks' time but has just been diagnosed with syphilis. The community where she lives usually, called us and it was up us to hunt her down. It is to our great credit that we all share the responsibility to find the women when we need to. There is a fine line of patient confidentiality to walk, so it is primarily from midwife to midwife to RNS nurses. If this fails, we then ask the Aboriginal Liaison Officers, who usually track them easily. From there, we learn which town they have gone to. Natalia had gone to Halls Creek for sorry business. This is a wake/funeral and can take many days. It is understood that getting a woman to come to a hospital during this time is not likely. We were anxious to get Natalia treated for her STI to offer protection to her unborn baby. An underlying low iron level was also complicating her condition, so arrangements were made with the Halls Creek Hospital for her to attend for both treatment of syphilis and get an iron infusion.

Sorry business and then disbursement of royalties meant she didn't attend.

However, the bush telegraph was working, and Natalia arrived in the hospital. Last-minute negotiations with the PATS team ramped up, and I was, for the second time, out at the airport. Natalia was on her way to Derby on the mail plane. She had her mobile phone and a plastic bag with a pair of jandals in it. The mail plane is a small twin-engine craft that flies every day between Broome Derby, Fitzroy Crossing and Halls Creek return.

Any of these women may put themselves on the bus and come home to Fitzroy. The system doesn't permit them to birth on in country, meaning where they live, nor does it finance a family member to accompany them when they go to sit down.

It is a white fellas' rule.

The third woman is Georgina, who works for an aboriginal organisation in the crossing. She has a screening ultrasound booked for the next day. She has a small bag packed and is at the hospital early. She, too, is booked on the mail plane. Georgina is a tall and strong woman. She is pregnant for the first time and is very excited. Her partner works in the town. They both live with his parents, who are also in Fitzroy crossing. They are one of the non-drinking families.

In my experience as a midwife, I have found that few indigenous mothers take responsibility for themselves, so it is refreshing and hopeful to see someone like Georgina show interest. However, I can't help but feel frustrated, empathetic, and even angry when trying to engage with pregnant women and try to make a small difference in their lives. As a transient midwife, I am limited in my ability to reach out to them or the system and people are fractured. The weight of the past is hindering progress, and while I do my best, it can feel like it's not enough for now.

At the end of that day, I had an unfamiliar feeling of accomplishment. I had been to the airport four times to either collect colleagues or drop off clients. I had seen a charter school plane taking aboriginal students based near Tunnel Creek, to Victoria for their next term of education. I had seen the RFDS plane return a man with his leg amputated. Drugs were delivered, and Lab specimens were exchanged. When it all works, it all works. That particular day I had seen more examples of aircraft than I had ever seen before. Twin engine Cessna, twin-turboprop, Bombardier Dash 8-100 Cessna, Caravan tiny two-seater helicopter, bigger six-seater helicopter, RFDS craft, and top dressing plane. It was as though FX was the centre of the universe.

The airport had a gate with the punch code 1 1 1 1 1 – we all knew it. The terminal was like a bus shelter with a bench seat. On one end, someone had written Domestic, the other International.

The Fitzroy Crossing airport was a vibrant spot.

37 GOOD FRIDAY FITZROY CROSSING

Once again, Easter had arrived, and I couldn't help but reflect on the past year. It was around this time last year that I was in quarantine in Alice Springs, trying to adjust to the pandemic's sudden changes. I vividly remember watching the Andrea Bocelli concert live stream, feeling a sense of connection to the rest of the world as the streets lay empty in cities around the globe. However, the drone shot of my usual shopping spot in London's Crouch End haunted me, and it was a sobering reminder that I was still in Australia, far from the life I used to know.

Throughout the pandemic, air travel had become limited, unreliable, and uncertain. As the virus surged and receded with the changing seasons in the northern hemisphere, I constantly considered the idea of returning to London. "I'm going back to London," I would repeat to myself, like a mantra or a safety rope. However, I was in a constant state of conflict, torn between making the most of my work as a midwife in rural Australia and longing for my old life that was slowly but surely eroding away. I would plan to travel at the end of my contract, but every time a new surge hit Europe, my plans were thwarted, and I would take on another contract. Meanwhile, my friends back home were adjusting to a new way of life, working from home, or not working at all, with limited travel even within their cities. Our conversations were dominated by the virus, and while I knew I was lucky to have work, I didn't feel it. Even though my children urged me not to come back, saying it was "shit" back home, or to stay and keep working and travelling, I still felt torn and conflicted.

I watched, listened, and lived the pandemic as a voyeur from the seemingly coronavirus-free Australia.

So here I was a year on, in Fitzroy Crossing. I reminded myself to make every day count.

My colleague at work said, *"Teresa, with a name like yours, there must be some Catholic in you? Do you want to come to the Stations of the Cross for Good Friday, tomorrow?"*

This was out of the blue but not as much of a surprise as learning Fitzroy Crossing had a Catholic Church. My Catholic days were well put to sleep since my divorce, and I accepted the invite out of sheer curiosity.

From the outside, St Francis Catholic Church looked neither like a house nor a church except for the roof line that pyramids upwards, extending to a slim cross that is faintly visible against the blue sky. Painted yellow, it is a steel clad space with regular windows and three garage doors. Each door is secured by one bolt inside and a hinge-pulley system which makes for easy operation. When opened, outside and inside blend, the ceiling fans swirl the humid air. On a good day the easterly breeze calms the heat.

I arrived just at 10:00 as directed. As I went inside, Miriam, dressed in shorts and t-shirt, was opening and closing cupboards, and Astha Aster, a children's health nurse, was sorting through CD'S. No one else was there. I wondered if I had gotten the time wrong. Miriam was flustered.

When I had arrived in Fitzroy Crossing, Miriam was thrilled to see me. "You were my mentor back in 2006 when I was a student midwife. Derby days," she said. She showered me with very kind accolades and said that I was instrumental in helping her pass the training. She also said that she was delighted that I had arrived in FX as she knew I was a very knowledgeable midwife."

I vaguely remembered Miriam, but the imposter syndrome kicked in, and I started doubting my current knowledge compared to what I knew back then. After all, it had been a long time since the Derby days, and the memories were a bit daunting. Nevertheless, I knew that Miriam had stayed in FX and was still working there. She had never remarried and spent her holidays visiting her son in Queensland. Miriam was involved in many community groups, including the volunteer fire service and indigenous liaison groups. She seemed to know everyone in town and everything about the community health service. She came across as competent but overworked and overtired, like an old-time professional who had been on the job for too long.

She was "always going to leave". I heard through the midwifery bush telegraph that she went on holiday not long after I had left and never came back.

It seems to be the way of it when you work in such testing conditions.

Neither the politicians nor the Australians have any fecking idea what the outback towns and communities are really like

"I have to pop home to get something," Miriam said...there's water in the fridge; help yourself, I won't be long."

With that, she left.

Aster too urgently remembered something she needed, and said,

"Can you mind the church? I've just got to pop home. I'll put the CD on. Won't be long."

After this flurry of activity, I was left standing in the middle of the room, minding the church, whatever that meant, listening to American folk Christian singing bellowing out from the CD player.

I felt that I had somehow been caught on candid camera or left in a scene from The Truman Show.

The fridge was in the back room, so I poured myself a glass of water, came back into the space, and sat looking around and taking it all in.

It was easy to imagine the old times with large congregations gathering. I doubt there were gospel singers or handheld fans, perhaps a mix of Aboriginal Aunties in bright frocks and families from the stations. This is outback Australia. The space felt colonised. A purple Saturn cloth covered the crucifix, the tabernacle had been opened and the consecrated hosts removed to the small but secure cupboard out the back. Strategically placed around the church were the twelve stations of the cross, identifying this space as a catholic church. Each native timber cross was numbered with roman numerals. Below each one was an aboriginal-styled depiction of the journey Jesus made, from trial to resurrection, painted on a small canvas. They were beautiful pieces of art.

I felt calm and contemplative until "Jesus loves you, Jesus loves you Jesus loves you," kept repeating from the scratched CD. Suddenly it was all a bit much for this once Catholic, agnostic midwife.

Who actually uses CDs anyway, I thought as I switched the player off at the wall.

Another flurry of activity commenced.

Miriam arrived back first, this time wearing a dress and muttering about not being able to find the lovely wee books that have the stations in them.

Then she lost her phone. "Should I phone it?" I offered. She was so distracted, she didn't reply and just left for home to find it.

Aster then returned, and Marcella arrived. I was introduced to Marcella from Mauritius. She was the town physio's wife. She wore a white trouser suit, cool cotton and draping. Her sunglasses were designer, she had make-up on, and wore a golden clasp to keep her long hair up off her collar.

Aster and Marcella knew each other and struck up a conversation about the stations. I saw my nursing colleague in a whole new light. Aster worked with children and was methodical and popular. We knew her as Aster, but she had a very eastern European name, and I was warned never to call her this. Aster was a single lady, but she shared her story with me one day. She had been married, and she had been pregnant 'too many times.' Her last pregnancy loss was at 24 weeks. Her husband left after that time. Aster sewed beautiful child-friendly uniforms to wear with pockets and places for all her toys and tools of the trade. Most of her visits involved immunisations. She had a wealth of distraction devices.

Today however, I saw Aster in a new light. I listened with incredulity as she claimed that, "When I listened to the stations, you know on my app, I have to stop when Jesus is nailed to the cross."

Her face was distorted with angst as she spoke, and she was wringing her hands in despair. "Oh, but I know Jesus had to do it for us, but oh, it is such an awful way to die."

"Yes, yes," Marcella nodded and agreed. "It's so very powerful, isn't it?"

Now I felt like I was in a freak show but couldn't walk out.

Meanwhile, Miriam had arrived back with her phone in her hand and set about synching the stations of the cross-app to the iPad via Bluetooth.

Asta and Marcelle offered to help. "There," said Miriam, she got it set to start.

"I'll just go and get Hanne. There's water in the fridge," she reminded us as she disappeared for the third time.

Marcella excused herself from Asta who was still fiddling around with the iPad, and offered me a drink. It was very hot, and it was only 10:30.

I grabbed my empty cup as Marcella was checking in the fridge. "Better not drink the holy water," she said, closing the door and opening a cupboard filled with small bottles and cans. "Would you like a Fanta?"

Oops! I thought. "Yes, thanks," I replied, not daring to disclose that I had already had two glasses of water from the fridge.

I had quite enjoyed the holy water. I felt blasphemous. Somehow I didn't think any of the three in this congregation would laugh.

Hanne, an elderly Aboriginal woman dressed in a floral skirt and long-sleeved cotton shirt, arrived and was helped with her Zimmer frame. Miriam was in her element, fussing and enabling.

I learned later that Hanne was the artist who had painted the stations. They were beautiful.

All assembled. 11 O'clock. Ready for kick-off I thought.

Then the iPad wouldn't play through the speakers that Miriam had laboured over earlier. I think Aster pushed a few too many buttons when she was playing the god songs.

With restrained annoyance, in the presence of god, I thought, Miriam and Aster both agreed to play the glorious mysteries of the cross via their respective app at the same time.

I knew that was never going to work – it's like having two devices playing the same radio station in a home. There is always a lag of some minuscule time.

And so after much ado, the glorious mysteries of Stations of the Cross, Good Friday at St Francis catholic church in Fitzroy Crossing commenced.

The seating arrangements were such that the five of us sat in a row; we didn't do the traditional walk from station to station. I sat between the two iPads, Marcelle beside Aster, and Hanne beside Miriam.

An intercessory response was to be sung intermittently in a Southern American accent. Cats choir is what came to mind. I felt a strange mix of incredulity and hysteria building.

After ten minutes of hell, it finished.

Miriam invited me to the Easter Sunday mass. The priest was coming for 7 pm service, she said. A flash of curiosity of what kind of priest would bother to come to Fitzroy Crossing passed through me.

"Thank you for asking me, but I've something else on," I lied.

38 WANGKATJUNGKA CLIENTS

Another day in the life of a remote community midwife.

Remote midwifery in Australia is as far removed from central London midwifery as you can imagine. Since the brutal rape and murder of a remote nurse a few years ago, protocols dictate that we never travel to communities alone and have on-call support. This is especially so for RANS nurses who live in remote communities. This came about after the passage of a bill in the South Australian Parliament, "Gayle's Law," in November 2017.

I joined the nursing team in the work 4x4 high clearance Toyota to go to one of our remote communities. During my placement in FX, each week, I would travel to Wankajonka, and without fail, some surprise would await me.

Like the time I discovered the family of redback spiders on the outside frame of our carport at the clinic. When I say family, it was more like a tribe. Over the weekend, the little critters had cooked up a storm of a web, a quite disorganised web, a nursery for a new batch of their offspring. There seemed to be only one big spider, a few medium sized, and zillions of dots of growing spiders. It was the big one that caught my eye. I hadn't actually had an encounter with a redback[1] before.

I cringed at myself as I said to my colleague, "Are you sure they are redbacks? How do you know?" Duh. Not much imagination is necessary as they have an obvious red/orange stripe on their shiny black abdomen and an hourglass spot on the underside. Even I could see it and knew exactly what breed it was. I don't know how dangerous they are, but the redback on the toilet seat song from my childhood assured me they could kill. Cool as a cucumber, my colleague phoned the pest man and assured me that they would be dealt with by the end of the week. What exact week she was referring to, I've no idea. Getting things done in the outback is a fluid timeframe and will always require patience. She also got a can of pest spray and dealt with them directly. I felt mildly reassured.

The community is 130 kilometres south-east of Fitzroy Crossing. There are about 180 permanent residents, Wangkatjungka, Walmajarri or Gooniyandi, with strong links to their desert culture. There is a store, health clinic, playgroup, school, and administration office, including a community hall and kitchen. There is, of course, also a footy ground.

Driving out to the clinic, it's a partial highway and then a graded gravel road, with small signs to direct the traveller. The landscape is dry, and it is hot in summer. There are plenty of waterholes and caves close by if you know where to go.

As you get closer to the community, the school is the first building you see. It is secured by high fences, and freshly painted in blue with local art on the walls. There is secure staff housing neatly kept and which is quite a contrast to what you see as you enter the community along the street. Here you will be met by the starkness of houses, derelict cars, rubbish, tyres, and dogs. The roads are dirty and busy with people walking about, especially if the shop is open. It has set opening hours, and it's a good place to find clients if they are needed at the clinic.

As a visitor to their community, it is normal for me to only see things on a superficial level. As you spend time, as some of my colleagues have done, you are exposed to the cultural depths and contradictions. It is reported that six out of ten white Australians have had little or no contact with aboriginal people. Out of those that have, I can only guess that maybe one would have ever been to a community. For this alone, I feel privileged.

It is impossible to enter an indigenous community and not be shocked, challenged, and forever affected by what you see. Each time is confronting. Each time I'm conflicted as I meet the women from the country. Behind closed doors, there are more differences than similarities to any other pregnant woman I've worked with. Their needs are more complex, and their expectations more simple. The more time I spend with them, the more I feel we are meeting their needs on their terms in such a small way. They are expected to fit into our midwifery guidelines, our timetables, to have their births in towns and have their care from us white fellas.

There is a gap that is getting bigger. But for now, I bring my cultural awareness, born in Aotearoa, New Zealand, my experience in midwifery and parenting, and my professionalism that needs to be adapted to community settings.

Many women have left an imprint on my midwifery soul. Marshya is one.

One Thursday, I had arranged to meet with three mums living there, and I took all the notes I thought I might need. Many families travel between the different communities, so it could easily happen that a pregnant mother I've never met would call to see me. If I don't have her hand-held records, I know the information I have will be patchy.

When I arrived, the mum who was to have her glucose testing done was in Fitzroy Crossing. This happens with monotonous regularity, and I accept this as part of the challenge of providing care to remote women. I know she will get the test done when it suits her.

Meanwhile, one of our other mums was waiting for the clinic to open. This generally means something is bothering them.

Marshya was thirty one weeks with her fourth baby. Her first and third babies had been born by caesarean section. She had complex medical issues, including labile hypertension, gestational diabetes, syphilis, and kidney disease. This is not that unusual for our clients.

Most of our indigenous women are shy. She had a trusting relationship with my colleague so my first job was to let her know that she had left.

When I accepted the position at Fitzroy Crossing, I was informed I would be the second midwife. Jane had been there for some months. On my arrival, I met my colleague very briefly at the end of the first day. She had been out at one of our remote communities, and so it wasn't until the next morning we got a chance to talk.

"Lets go for coffee," she said, "Its better to get away, or we won't be left alone."

Fitzroy has a newish coffee shop run by the local indigenous corporation. There the staff are offered training and work experience. It has great coffee too.

Jane, similar age to me, is tall and wiry. We had a very brief exchange of our journey to Fitzroy Crossing and got down to business. I sensed anxiety in Jane. She remained professional, and we started what would be a short but wonderful working relationship.

The child health nurse, with whom I had developed a positive rapport, had persistently bothered Jane, causing unnecessary obstacles in her work life. These obstacles included difficulties with her accommodations and barriers with our nursing colleagues. Jane didn't disclose all of the details to me and instead utilised the appropriate channels of complaint through the line managers. Unfortunately, FX had a chain of line managers, none of whom were able to provide support for Jane.

Shortly after, a male nurse who had previously worked in elder care at FX, joined as our new manager. I had been working for three weeks when an intense argument erupted between Ata and Jane. Ata had no reservations about verbally abusing Jane, who remained composed and professional throughout the incident. The following day, Jane handed over her list of clients to me and abruptly left her job. At the time, I was unaware that I would soon become the next target.

Back at the clinic I greeted Marshya. "It's lovely to see you," I said. "I suppose you would have been expecting Jane, but she has left Fitzroy and asked me to send her goodbyes and wish you a happy, happy birth."

She gave me an almost imperceivable nod to say she understood.

"How are you feeling today?"

"A little bit alright," she said quietly

This confirms that something is bothering her.

"Can you tell me what has happened?"

"I got some wet stuff. I think it might be my waters breaking. It's a little bit early."

She looked at me, and I knew she understood that this was not supposed to be happening.

"Have you felt your little baby moving this morning?"

She nodded.

"That's a really good start." I smiled at her.

"Let's have a look and see what's happening," I said

And so the morning started off in that oh-so-unexpected way.

Immediately I had to step into obstetric emergency mode; assess, diagnose and negotiate through a new system of transferring this mother to a hospital for safe delivery. One of the nurses working at the clinic was on a graduate programme and was with me learning a "bit of midwifery." She got to witness first-hand how challenging and urgent some situations can be.

I've been involved in such transfers, but never from a remote setting. The clerk at the Royal Flying Doctors Service (RFDS), where we phone directly, was calm, triaged the situation, and then transferred my call to the operations Doctor. From here, he took a detailed history and, at each step, commended and affirmed that we had done the appropriate care. He was calm and certainly a reassuring voice for me at the end of the telephone.

With RFDS in action, I continued the initial treatments to halt the labour and expedite transfer, catheterise and examine the cervix, gain IV access, provide antibiotic cover and prepare her for flight to Perth.

This shy, but savvy mum, was quiet throughout the procedures. It was all hands on deck, and we chatted and reassured her, explaining each step as it was performed. There were plentiful phone calls, paperwork, and observations of mum and her unborn baby.

The logistics required dispatching an ambulance with a doctor to come from Fitzroy. This round trip would take just under four hours. I would accompany the ambulance to FX airport, where I would hand over to the RFDS team, who would fly the one hour flight to Broome, where the jet and crew would then fly the mother to Perth airport and the ambulance transfer to King Edward Memorial Hospital.

By 4 pm, with impressive precision, including emptying the catheter bag onto the airport grass, it was job done for me as we waited until the plane had taken off.

I found it difficult to explain how I felt. With more than eight weeks before the due date, this woman had been plucked out of her home and community. My colleague Miriam, whom all the locals loved and knew, had to go to her home to collect her clothes and purse. She really wanted to get her own belongings. Even this was not possible.

Her mum and then the boyfriend arrived to say goodbye. All through this, she was quiet.

She was settled into the back of the ambulance, and as we drove past the community school where two of her children were in their classrooms, I saw the sadness on her face and a wee tear trickle down.

"Are the others at school today?" I asked.

"Yes, they are there. I didn't say goodbye. They'll be wondering why I'm not there to pick them up."

I realised right then that although it had been busy and time-constrained to get (this young mum's name) to Perth, I had not acknowledged her other children.

"I'm so sorry," I said.

"They'll be alright; their dad will pick them up," she said.

They would not see their mum for many weeks.

In the back of the ambulance, I gave her my corned beef sandwich I had made that morning, and we shared an orange. It was the first food she had had that day.

Marshya's baby was born by emergency C section within 23 hrs of her presenting to our clinic.

This indigenous woman with obstetric and medical complexities that should never exist in a woman of childbearing years; yet she intuitively knew to come to get help, and I am so glad I was there for her that day. If I do nothing much else in my time here, I've made a difference, I thought. Even though at the end of the day, I'm just doing my job.

Against the odds, this woman is a survivor. Her life is one of survival. What amazing intuition. I'm in awe of her.

The women from Fitzroy Crossing were more transient than in other places I had worked. There seemed to be more sorry times. All symptoms of a fractured community. When Marysha arrived back in the community two months after having been air lifted to Perth, no health professionals were aware she had returned.

An alert had been emailed with the baby's name, which did not have any reference to the mother's name. It was the newborn history and gestation of the baby that alerted Asta Aster, the CHN, that it was Marshya. Mother, along with her newborn had slipped through the postnatal system. Mother had been discharged from KEMH[2] and missed her postnatal midwifery visits because she was spending time with her baby in SCBU (Special Care Baby Unit). She arrived back in the community without her essential hypertension medication, no follow-up of her kidney failure, or her syphilis serology. When the baby had been discharged from SCBU in Perth, mum and baby had been referred to Broome paediatric care; however, upon arrival, they had been turned away and stayed in a hostel because there were no spare beds. Mum and baby caught the first bus out of Broome and got a lift to their remote community, where I accidentally saw them the day I went out. Meanwhile, they had been lost in the paperwork/email system.

I despair. On the surface, a few simple changes could have made a big difference. If the midwifery service had a generic email that any services across WA could access, if they had not been turned away from a hospital, if the FX provided a safe workspace for the midwife, so there was not such a turnover of staff, on and on it goes... round and round and round.

As it happened, Marshya came to see me and to show me her beautiful wee baby. She was so happy to be home, reunited with her three older children and family. Despite my many phone calls to the Perth Social Work department, this mum never had anyone with her during her birth and weeks in SCBU. She said they always said they would arrange it, but it never happened.

On reflection, it seems a happy ending, mum and baby both well and safely home. But in reality, one more indigenous woman was plucked from country and family, birthed on her own over 2500km away, and was almost lost in a system when she was spat out of the city hospital. All is not well.

My stern words to Marshya were that she had to speak up and speak out. She needs to gather the other beautiful young women from her community and somehow stop this isolation during birth. It upsets me deeply knowing that, with all the money that is thrown at the indigenous communities, the simple cost to have your birth partner or sister/ mother with you as a support is denied to so many.

39 ANZAC DAY 2021

As a child growing up in New Zealand (now known also as Aotearoa), Anzac Day was the day my dad would pin his medals left side of his chest, and march with the Veterans greeting the dawn to commemorate the loss and significance of the sons and daughters who fought and died in the wars. He was a Korean war vet. Anzac day is a much revered public holiday in Australia and New Zealand.

My earliest Anzac memory is attending the Dawn Service at the Invercargill Cenotaph, where my Big Brother BB was in his ATC uniform standing (reverse arms whats the stance) holding a rifle. I would have been six years old.

In 2014, I was part of the Ngati Ranana Hikoi/ journey to Messines, Flanders in Belgium, which is part of the western front, where we were to partake in the opening of the Messines Museum and the unveiling of the New Zealand soldier, who appears in photos of the pilgrims who visit the western front every year. During this excursion, I started my journey of awareness about the plight of our soldiers who came from the utmost corners of the earth to battle. Each year, I would return to the Western Front, an easy journey from London, but here I was in the back of beyond. But I was buoyed to know that even in Fitzroy Crossing, there would be a dawn service.

I had to push aside the hanging disbelief that I was still in Australia.

The sun was awakening to a beautiful day, the dry season now not sweltering hot at 5:30. At the visitor's centre, three Australian flags and one from New Zealand adorned the entrance flanking the 'Lest We Forget' sign and the Australian Rising Sun emblem strung across the entrance.

The coordinator, a Colombian immigrant new to the Kimberley, did a fantastic job organising and partaking in her first-ever Anzac service. I'm sure she will always remember this day.

About a hundred local residents, police, boy scouts, soldiers from Derby, and locals gathered, welcomed to the country and remembered the ANZAC's, and all who serve in the defence force. I read a piece of prose I'd written for the Ngati Ranana 60th anniversary visit to the Western Front.[1]

Jess, a Kiwi teacher, and I had said we would brave it and sing the NZ anthem, but neither of us are actual singers. We thought in a small crowd, no one would notice. As the numbers grew, I got a tad nervous and hoped like hell Jess could hold a note. We both spotted a tall Maori fella wearing a New Zealand Rugby league warriors t-shirt. Jess went and persuaded him to join us, which he reluctantly did. We had the lyrics already prepared and on the programme so it was all good.

Along with a scattering of other Kiwis, we sang our national anthem in Te Reo Maori and English as a helicopter flew by, lifting our eyes to the skies and providing a perfect distraction from the amateur choir.

A sausage sarnie breakfast followed. The only thing missing was a tot of rum – a tradition from my numerous Anzac days in Ypres, not possible in this 'dry community.'

I had now been in Australia by accident for two Anzac days.

When working in rural or remote communities, we depend on

strangers to be our friends. I call them situational friends. They are people whose path you would not ordinarily cross, and in many instances, will not do after your situation changes.

"Anyone want to come on a tiki tour?" asked Jess. Eimer, who had recently arrived in FX, and who was living in my old digs 'big brother house, asked what a tiki tour was.

"It's like a Sunday drive, but without a destination," she said. "If you have nothing better to do today, come with us, and you will find out."

Eimer was not convinced but willing to join the banter, and the promise of a swim in the cool outdoors was an opportunity not to be missed.

Ruth, too, joined us. She confessed she had been too shy to join us up the front singing but assured us she sang in the crowd.

As it happened, we did get to the quarry for a swim just as the sun was setting. A perfect end to an inspirational day.

Jess, our driver, has been in Fitzroy Crossing FX for a few years, having left her life in NZ penniless and still mourning the loss of financial security, lavish lifestyle, and meaningful employment. She was not mourning the loss of her second husband. She came as a cook to a station, slowly healed her wounds, and was now back teaching. She is a horsewoman and spends time and money caring for her nag and being grannie to two Derby-born grandchildren.

Toyota Hilux is a common vehicle here in the Kimberley's and, unlike the yummy mummies of Highgate, used for its intended purpose. Off-road and back-country driving.

Ruth, a dialysis nurse, was once a midwife and had Irish and English family connections. She has been a *fly in fly out* (FIFO) nurse for years. She had been in FX for three months and, because of short staffing, had spent most of her time working double shifts. This was her first time in the Kimberley region and her first trip out of town. Two of her daughters are pregnant, so she thinks this will be her last season. She is well healed following her divorce and emotional extraction from a violent relationship.

Eimer is a freshie to remote. She is Irish-born and adopted Australia as her country over forty years ago. She is here to run the coronavirus vaccine clinic. Eimer has not been out of WA and is seldom even out of Perth. The situational contrasts have been quite confronting during her first three weeks. Unhappily married, she described the joy she felt when she had to have her wedding band cut off after a bicycle accident and suffered a broken finger. She is exploring the possibility of "independence" from a life partner who she now dislikes. There is bubbling emotion below the surface, but she is a Catholic. Eimer's three children are independent, and one has recently had a baby, so she too is a grandmother.

I was the networker who knew the three other women. They were strangers to each other. This was a tiki tour that could be interesting.

It was 8 am, and the sun was already in full sight, heating the day. With a good breakfast of patriotism and sausage sarnie, we headed west along the highway, then turned north, ignoring the "road closed" sign. Jess thought it might be interesting to see how the road was after the wet season. I wondered out loud if we could go to Tunnel Creek. We drove slowly over rather rutted roads, through shallow flowing streams, stopping to photograph the beef stock (not the powdered variety for soup) and the changing landscape. Eimer was agog at the scenery. The wonder of the Kimberley's never leaves us but having a freshie amongst us reminded me of my first time seeing the boab trees, wild beasts, and the drama of colour as the rock formations arise like a golden mountain statue, to honour the ancestors of this land. Jess acted as a tour guide and drove into an abandoned station that had just had a lease renewal.

"There will be Wagyu beef herds thumping through this land before we can catch the photo of a Tatar Lizard," our driver said. They will join the healthy-looking Brahman we pass today roaming free, casting their wary eye on our vehicle.

The road we are on is a popular dry-season road to Windjana Gorge, part of the infamous Gibb River Road tourist route. About 80km in, there is a school. Seemingly in the middle of nowhere, it is called Yiramalay/Wesley Studio school. Like an oasis in the desert, its principles are a welcome concept to a troubled Aboriginal story. The Studio School is founded on an equal partnership between two diverse cultures and communities: the Bunuba people of Fitzroy Valley and Wesley College in Melbourne. The Studio School is said to deliver *life-changing learning experiences that transcend culture and location*. It was these students I had seen being flown out of their community during the floods recently. We drove through the campus and saw tidy and well-presented facilities, including outdoor school rooms under the shade of canvas. The grounds had been watered by bore water and provided beautiful green outdoor spaces.

Wondering how much further Tunnel Creek might be, we stopped and had a yarn with a couple in a white utility vehicle coming towards us. It's what people do on this road; just stop and have a yarn, very like on the roads in the Burren Co. Clare, Ireland.

Jess wound down the window and said, "Gidday, how far to Tunnel Creek?

The aboriginal driver dressed in his station work clothes of wrangler jeans, checked long-sleeved shirt, and Akubra hat didn't need to wind down his window because there wasn't even a door. I stared at the 'flintstones' car in awe. It took him a while to respond.

I figured he had heard the question in English, translated it to Creole, then asked his partner in their language before answering.

There was an ambiguous reply. "*A little bit* further," he said. "*Not too far. Youllbealright.*"

The couple both had beautiful smiles and waved us goodbye. I feared for them if they were to go onto the main road. No seat belts either.

Tunnel Creek was in fact a further 30km on and over a rough road. We bumped and swerved over rocks and dried mud, following other tyre marks along spinifex grass edges or off-road to avoid deep hollows. Jess negotiated our vehicle around even deeper ruts as the lands evolved from pasture to picturesque, the steep red rocks heralding Tunnel Creek.

We put together our picnic and then explored the gorge. There may be freshies in the tunnel, Jess warned. They are similar to salties but have long, narrow snouts and don't usually attack humans. Eimer nodded. I was not convinced. Only then Eimer realized we were talking about crocodiles.

Unseasonal clear water was still flowing through the tunnel, and we slipped and hopped over the rocks as far as was safe to negotiate. The water and red sand swallowed up my jandal. I'm optimistic it will be spat out and there for me when I return with my Kiwi buddy, Jeff in June.

The highlight of this tiki tour was not the wildlife nor the majestical scenery but the stories that four women, relative strangers, shared. For eight hours, almost competing for talk time, we made connections between towns in Ireland and New Zealand. We talked about places and people we knew and shared stories. Jess and Ruth Ruth were both working in Christchurch hospital when the disastrous earthquake hit on 22nd February 2011, so we learned first-hand of their horrific day. I found this so very sobering. I had been in London with my four adult kids and husband at the time, all celebrating my 50th birthday. We got home just after midnight to the news. Christchurch had been our home before we left to live in Ireland in 2003.

There were multiple Irish connections amongst us all, through Counties Tipperary and Cork. We gossiped and laughed about our former husbands and confessed our guilty secrets - thoughts of ways we had considered getting rid of them. Eimer initially feigned shock, then added to the conspired ideas. From stabbing to suffocation, willing a diver not to surface, and simple gunshot, we all shared our stories, and I believe the relief was palpable. To date, none of us needed to carry out any such acts. All we needed to do was work in rural and remote Australia.

There was talk about sex or lack of it, self-pleasuring toys, and where Eimer could buy her first one from. We compared birth stories, and the two grannies talked of the fine line it is to let our kids go; yet will them to make good parenting choices. We talked of money, its loss, and the discrepancies in wages in rural towns. We all agreed that $2200 per day was unfair.

It's what doctors get paid in Fitzroy Crossing.

The remote services in Australia are full of women like the four in the vehicle that day. Australia has a road map for strong independent nurses, midwives, and teachers, many of whom step away from their former lives and strive to gain emotional healing and financial independence.

Some don't make it. Many do. Situational friendships help the process.

It is also a place where life long friends are made.

As it happened, we did get to the quarry for a swim just as the sun was setting. A perfect end to an inspirational day.

Settling into my new accommodation was easy. Having initially not wanted to share with some crazy misfit colleague (this is what I imagined and have had experienced before) I shared the space with Wendy, a Londoner originally who had lived in NZ and had two Kiwi born daughters. Wendy spoke so candidly of her delightful life in a wee town called Rawene. I had not heard of it. She played the ukulele and was a well-respected returnee staff nurse to the crossing. We have remained friends. All was mostly going well except for the frogs.

Fx Needs a Frog Warning

Frogs are a common sight in FX. Not to be confused with the cane toads that were introduced into Queensland and are making their way across Australia's top end(via Fitzroy crossing). Those horrid beasts have no natural enemies and devastate native animal species and ecosystems. The Fitzroy frogs are smaller, about the size of an apricot, bright green, and live in trees AND and in my toilet, apparently.

They are persistent. They are plentiful. The first time I encountered one clinging to my screen door, I took photos and admired its cuteness. They have padded Velcro-like pads as feet and can spring and cling with acrobatic dexterity.

The next encounter was not so welcome or so cute.

It was 2 am in the morning. With low lights and no footwear, I made my way to the loo. Luckily for both the frog and me, I glanced into the toilet bowl before sitting. In a moment of terror I Instinctively flushed, hoping the green monster would be down the pipes before either of us knew what was happening. But as the swirling water from the cistern settled, it was still there, clinging to the toilet bowl. I witnessed a frog's desperate attempt at survival, his four legs stretched across the porcelain, clinging on as the torrent of water failed to detach them. As the flow stopped, the green cling-on leapt vertically up onto the lid, then onto the wall right past my head, bouncing higher up the wall, down the door, and onto the floor.

By this stage, I was yelling at it; what I was yelling, who knows (maybe the neighbours might know).

I was scared witless, and my adrenalin was pumping.

I had a flashback from many years ago when I still had a phobia of birds - something I eventually overcame. Back then, I found a hen in the sunporch pecking around under my baby bassinet while my baby lay sleeping. So like that day when I caught the chicken, I knew I had to be brave and catch the frog.

I found nurses' gloves and some paper towels. By this time, the frog was in the kitchen and had leapt from the bench to the stovetop. I planned the operation in my head. I opened the ranch slider and unlocked the screen door – mindful that I didn't want anything worse coming in at night like more frogs or a snake.

Froggy was sitting on the back left element of the stovetop. I threw the paper towel over him and, before I could think too much, picked him up – paper and all and wrapped him in my gloved hand. I could feel convulsions like muscles and legs trying to escape, and I calmed my anxiety with a self-affirming message, "Its just a frog. You've got this."

Armed with this paper towel-wrapped glove encased frog, I stepped outside and, with Olympian determination, threw the bundle up and over the fence like an overarm shot put.

The cushioned thud of it hitting the neighbour's tin roof, although not intended, made me feel both awful and relieved.

The next day my Kiwi nurse colleague Lynda came bearing gifts of toilet blue and bleach. Even that didn't deter them. I started leaving toilet tissue in the loo as an added deterrent.

I've now gotten very used to checking under the rim and lids of the toilet and no longer have such a dramatic response to seeing the frogs. With wet gloved hands, I can pick the little monster up and place it on the front lawn for the hawkes to find. Eventually, I found out where they were getting in and with mepore tape from the hospital did an elaborate cover over the septic outlet pipe, leaving just enough gaps for air and not frogs.

I don't sleep easy. Years later, I still find myself checking the toilet before I sit.

My nightmares are of frogs with blue eyes and wet toilet tissue draping over their backs, the legs and sticky paws climbing up the bowl waiting for me at 2 am in the morning.

My friends are all laughing at me.

It's not funny.

40 CALLING IT A DAY

I've found during my times in remote and rural Australia, fellow New Zealanders, often by default perhaps, compare the plight of our indigenous populations in Aotearoa NZ to Australian First Nations people. Australians ask us about the differences. I find it so hard to explain to Ozzie's just how different it is. In Fitzroy's recent history, it is told that when the government changed the laws, as recently as 1969 - so that station owners had to pay the aboriginal workers equal money for their work, rather than just lodgings - the owners gathered up all the workers on the backs of their trucks or utility vehicles and dropped them into the towns of Halls Creek, Fitzroy crossing and Derby. The Kimberley people were likely affected by the government policies that resulted in the forced removal of First Nations children from their families, which is also known as the Stolen Generation. This practice continued until the 1970s.

I still find it hard to reconcile and imagine that this has actually happened during my lifetime.

The town of Fitzroy Crossing is widely known for its socioeconomic struggles, issues with alcohol abuse, and more recently, reports of unruly children. However, it's important to recognise that there's a deeper history of trauma and displacement behind these problems. During our work in Fitzroy Crossing, we noticed that most of our clients were descendants of indigenous peoples who were dispossessed and displaced. It's worth noting that these people were only officially recognised as part of the population in 1967, so only two generations later, their descendants were being born far from their ancestral lands and often on land that belonged to others. To make matters more complicated, many women were taken away from their families and transported to other towns to give birth.

I had met elder women from the stolen generation[1], many of whom are a stable and hopeful influence in the town. At some stage as a midwife, nurse, doctor, or teacher, it all becomes too much and takes an emotional and physical toll.

I had made a great network of friends in the Crossing. I learned to tolerate the frogs and avoid the spiders. I loved flying out in a caravan or turbo Cessna to Nookenbah every couple of weeks. I had started to network with the health promotions teams and were meeting women on the banks of the river for antenatal yarns. I loved the drive to Wankajonka with my nurse colleagues each Wednesday, and of course, I had begun to be trusted by the women.

I was becoming wary of our lack of management at work, and the unruly feral kids were concerning. I was becoming tired.

Jeff, my travel buddy, had been asking me to join him on a tiki tour of Australia's far north. His three month trip had been postponed the year before, and I had declined then, saying, "I'd love to, but I'm going back to London."

He had rescheduled due to Coronavirus, and again had asked me to join him, and my reply was the same. I thought of a plan, phoned him and said, "How about you come up to FX, and we do the Gibb River road? I can take a week of leave and then you can carry on with your trip, and I'll finish up my contract and head back to London. I thought this would be a great treat of a trip and would tide me over until my contract finished.

I arranged my annual leave and started to read up about the Gibb

River road trip. My flatmate Wendy and I would pour over the maps. She called it mapography, and said it was better than pornography. I got it.

After Jane, my colleague had left, the office administrator, having been reprimanded for her behaviour, had been better to work with. However, over time, her controlling and belligerent behaviours returned. Many workplaces have these obstructive clerical workers, but Ata's growing and obvious dislike of midwives blew up, and I was at the receiving end of a barrage of yelling abuse and accusations. It was as though a volcano had erupted in the corridors of the small wing of the Fitzroy Crossing Community health centre.

The child health nurse, heard the kerfuffle and closed her door, confiding later that she was scared and didn't know what to do. At the other end of the building, Miriam had heard it all and chose not to confront Ata directly but emailed the manager and included the WACHS (Western Australia Country Health Service) manager in the email. Disciplinary action followed, and Ata's contract was not renewed as she had assumed. She is no longer even in Australia.

For me, it was the last straw and a timely gift. I was shaken following the incident but got home, phoned Jeff and said, "You know how I was going to come on holiday with you for a week?" "Yes," he replied. "Well, I've resigned, and I'll come with you the whole way, is that ok?"

Yes, yes 100% yes he said, secretly thinking "Oh shit! I've got to put up with her for three months and get another camp stretcher".

My last shift was on a Thursday. Ata had taken leave, so it was a relief to not have to work with her that last shift. We had the compulsory farewell Prosecco and nibbles, with my gaggle of friends. Thibould, our new manager, confessed he too had already resigned after having had to deal with two episodes of office worker vs midwife dysfunction. My new friends met my travel buddy, and they all teased me about the 'friends status.' My reply was, "but he's my friend. We are travel buddies. We shared a hotel room in Switzerland, and after all, we are grown-ups and can share a bed and a tent."

What were they thinking?

The next morning, we loaded up the Trusty Toyota with my worldly possessions adding to Jeff's camping clobber, and left the crossing without a glance behind. It was the first time I had left a placement with such a palpable sense of relief. I would not to have to endure the misfits, missionaries and mercenaries who were battling against all odds to improve the health of the indigenous peoples, nor the out of control kids showing little signs of hope.

The freedom I felt was real. Three months of doing whatever we wanted and then I'd be back to London. Perfect I thought.

During our first couple of nights, we stayed with my cousin and celebrated their engagement. Cable Beach in Broome is a beautiful place to watch the sun and moon rising and setting. Locals swim there, but my imagination sees crocodiles, sharks, and stingers in the water, so I keep well away. Jenny and I, cousins both, enjoyed the rarity of time with family, sipped our Prosecco while the boys cooked the freshly caught fish on the barbie. For the first time in my life, I watched the moon disappear over the horizon, and as we waited for the night sky, Jenny said, "What could be more beautiful?" At that very moment, we both watched and caught a falling star.

That falling star might have been the magic sprinkled on Jeff and me.

Our first-night camping was just out of Derby, close enough so we could meet the plane that was to fly us to the Horizontal Falls[2] the following morning. We slipped into an easy travel buddy system, chatting, and planning with a comfort that only happens with friends. Both of us had discovered the Wikicamps App, and had similar thoughts about where we would prefer to camp.

Setting up the tent for the first time, Jeff had a good eye for the flattest spot, and the four-man pop up took only a few minutes. With the clear sky and warm temperatures we decided not to use the fly cover but to fall asleep under the southern cross. I set up the stretchers and bedding while Jeff gathered the wood and started the camp fire. We both put the dinner together.

"Here, cut the carrots this way," he said. I thought he was joking as he went to take the knife from me to demonstrate.

"Oh my god, you have been living alone way too long," I quipped, pointing the knife at him and then continuing to chop the veggies my way.

We laughed and enjoyed a delicious chicken and veggie dinner. The sun set early, and our evening was calm as we watched the embers dye off.

Jeff headed off track with a shovel, and I had a pee behind the car. I decided then and there that I couldn't be shy about dressing, toileting, and washing. After all, we were travel buddies, friends, and anyway we had met through outward bound where you strip off and shower with the whole watch of people.

The first night's view from our tent was of a boab tree, the moonlight reflecting on the branches cloaking its leafless limbs. The southern cross was not out just yet, but the milky way smeared her stars across the night sky.

I felt safe. I had left FX behind.

The Horizontal Falls experience was an indulgence we both had decided to do when I'd first arranged to have the five days together. What an experience. Float plane scenic flight over Derby, out over the archipelago and bird's eye view of the falls. Swimming with the sharks, jet boat through the falls and backwards and forward until the tide was too high. It was exhilarating and, as a tourist venture, perfectly executed. Fantastic food and photo opportunities ending with a scenic flight back to base.

We both talked about how wonderful it was to share this experience with someone else. I, too, had been single for too long.

My friend Jess, from FX had suggested we stay on her daughter's station, which had a boundary on Gibb River Road. The station is over 5,000 sq km or 1.2million acres.

The directions were specific, and we found the farm gate and billabong with daylight to spare. It was a beautiful piece of land. Jeff and I settled into our camp, setting up a routine (a system that was to continue throughout our whole trip) and within half an hour, the fire was blazing and the dinner was cooking.

"We can swim in the pond, apparently," I said. Jess had shown me photos of her and her horse cooling in the water.

"Will we have a wash in there?" I thought. Jeff would be keen, even though I secretly wasn't so.

"Or, we can have a bucket bath," he said. "I've got the hot water heating already."

"Much better idea," I agreed.

I'd made the decision not to be shy, so as Jeff fumbled with his clothes and towel, I stripped off and grabbed the soap.

I caught the look on his face. Surprise? Shock? Disbelief?

"We have got three months of this Jeff," I said, "We have just got to get used to it. I'll be buggered if I'm going to be hiding behind a towel while I have a bucket bath."

I realised that Jeff still hadn't said anything.

Jeff dropped his towel and reached for his washcloth.

I was very aware that I was naked in front of my friend and tried to act nonchalant, yet couldn't help but sneak a look at him. He did have a good body.

At that time, we both noticed his maleness had registered a naked female.

"Oi," I quipped.

Jeff covered himself, or should I say tried to cover himself, and we both started laughing.

We had positioned the tent to face East, not as a religious ritual but so we could see the sunrise. As the dawn chorus warmed up, the sun rose, first as cerise pink, maturing into a red, and then orange, it's arms stretching through the low-lying bushes. A mirrored reflection over the water captured by the frame of our tent window was a picture that we wanted to absorb. In silence, we watched the day waken, the colours change and lighten the essence of positivity and energy that nature shares willingly when we take the time to listen and watch.

I felt a change brewing within. I looked over at my travel buddy. He was so easy and fun to be around. I was happy, and I was relaxed. I realised that being in Australia by accident was taking its toll. For now, I could just be with nature. I didn't have to be a midwife; I could be myself.

Breaking the tranquillity and slapping me out of my daydreaming, there was a thunderous pounding of hooves as a mob of cattle appeared. I saw them heading directly towards our tent, but none came close as they veered off, leaving the water's edge, eventually stammering to a halt and busying themselves with grazing.

I poked my head out of the tent.

Jeff was up pottering away, sorting out the camp cooker. He seemed to enjoy watching the beasts, and I think he had a smile at my reaction.

"Don't worry, something just spooked them," said Jeff. He was in his element having come from a farming background. "They won't bother us." I did keep a wary eye on them from a distance though.

The billie was boiled and breakfast ready.

"Isn't this just the best? No work, warm weather, personal chef – a girl could get used to this," I teased.

"You're on dishes," he replied.

Jeff was tucking into his breakfast as I sipped my tea. The glorious thought of no work, the discovery of Australia; then for me it was back to London to pick up my life or pieces that were left, for Jeff it was for his return to Aotearoa New Zealand for a holiday initially, and then he was considering returning for good. Plans loosely conceived, yet to be executed.

We had no set agenda except a booking at the Hairy Dogs Fishing Camp near Wyndham at the end of the week. The Gibb River Road is a winter season adventure that you can drive in a day or take three months, stopping along the way to explore gorges with cool, clear water, aboriginal art, walks, and tourist experiences that during coronavirus were less frequent but at least bookable. The road was dirt, rough, and rutted at places. There were river crossings and road closures. There was a communal spirit and shared hints and advice. Jeff was in his element in his four wheel drive with a trusty co-pilot. It was fun.

When we pulled into Silent Grove, Jeff started his search for a flat area to set up camp. This is a popular campground, and dozens of interesting tents, vans, and home kit campers were already set up.

He found a space, parked the utility vehicle, and started unloading the gear.

Right in front of the area slithered a snake. About 1.5 metres long, slithery brown-black in colour.

"Oh shit, Jeff, there's a snake."

I've been in Australia long enough not to overreact like I used to, and I was impressed with my calmness.

We watched it slither from the reeds across our tent site near the camp building, and then it disappeared.

"He's gone. He won't bother us," said Jeff.

"But what if he's just gone to the shop and will come back?" I was trying to make light of the situation that we were about to set up camp in a snake pit.

"Just keep the tent zipped up and wear your shoes." A standard piece of advice.

"See! I yelled as the snake reappeared slithered back past our tent and then disappeared into the reeds."

When the ranger came around to collect the camp fees, I asked him,

"What happens if you get bitten by a snake?"

"Oh, well," he took his time answering, "you would have to come over to the warden's hut, and we would have to arrange a helicopter and all that." "We would have to get you out to a hospital pretty quickly, you know."

"So first aid is still pressure and immobilise?"

"Well, yes, that is what you do, but we are a long way away from help, really, and depending on the time of day and the weather, it's quite a business, so best you just don't get bitten by a snake."

"I just saw one," I said

"Oh, that's just Bob."

"Bob?"

"Yes, he lives here. He'll leave you alone. Just keep your tent zipped and wear your shoes."

"Where have I heard that before?" I mused.

Bob was the topic of conversation for a while as we met and shared stories with other campers. It really was a beautiful place to be staying.

Later that night, as we were safely zipped up in our tent, Jeff shyly said, " There's something I want to do. Can I kiss you?"

"I think I'd like you to," I said.

He leaned over from his stretcher. His two strong hands cupped my face, and he kissed me for a very long time.

The memory of the kiss lingered as a lightness during the next day. I tried not to analyse or anticipate what it meant. We found an exclusive campsite with abundant firewood. After our dinner that night, as the sun was setting and the moon was hanging in the sky, I quietly said to Jeff, "How about we continue where we left off last night?"

I slept that night with the twinkle of the stars through the tent, the moonlight glistening on the water, and cupid's arrow filling my chest with a feeling I had long forgotten.

What happens in the tent stays in the tent.

Except to say that for the next three months, we continued our journey in each other's close company day and night. We laughed, we walked, we explored, we made love, and we slept like angels. All through the magic of the Kimberley, across the border to Darwin, we explored and soaked up the knowledge and sunshine. We came across most of the wildlife Australia boasts of, we drove up a road that was officially deemed 'should not really be a road.' It was 33% steepness. We met colleagues I had met all over Australia and stayed with friends. Across the Gulf of Carpentaria to the far north Queensland we saw the plantations, and I learned that pineapples grow in the ground. Did anyone know that pineapples don't grow on trees? Jeff knew. You know what? I said, the only thing we haven't bought from a stall is pineapple. I'd love to buy a fresh pineapple". I wanted to buy a pineapple from a stall. There were many fresh produce stalls in the far north, and we had lived off fresh seasonal produce as much as we could.

I hadn't noticed particularly where we were heading, but as we turned up into a long driveway I asked Jeff where were we going. It's a surprise he said, just wait. It was then I saw the sign, painted on a pallet, "pineapples" with an arrow pointing to a large shed. We had pulled into a plantation – that's when I saw pineapples growing in the ground.

What are they?

Pineapples?

What?

Pineapples, Jeff replied again.

But they are in the ground! I said with incredulity. I really had led a sheltered life.

Way you go, said Jeff.

I was still trying to accept the reality that pineapples didn't grow in a tall palm like tree, like the tree outside my quarantine apartment in Alice Springs and were actually little plants at ground level. Going up to where the workers were packing and a little unsure if they actually sold to the public, I said to a Maori woman, "do you sell pineapples?"

She was holding a pineapple in each hand and said, "No, sorry, we only sell strawberries."

She got me.

Her smile won the day. "*Kia ora*," she said. "*Kia ora*," I replied.

Jeff had been laughing for a long time. He had heard it all. I got to try the three different varieties and in the end bought one of each.

They were delicious. I am still fascinated about my new knowledge about the humble pineapple.

The only time we slept in a bed was in a Port Douglas time share, where we dabbled our toes into domestic normality and continued our compatible journey being visitors to the area. The Whitsunday islands we decided was the most beautiful place in the world. We spent a day soaking in the picture perfect colours and silicone sands, snorkelling and swimming.

Almost a perfect day, apart from my enduring memory, and I imagine the tour guide may well be scarred for life as I returned to the boat after our time onshore for a lunch stop. Jeff already up on deck watched, laughing at (and with) me along with most of the other passengers. Jack, a wiry good looking young man, had to place both his hands on my ample arse, giving me a shove as I hoisted myself up. The boat was drifting away from the shore. Jack, very good-humouredly said " too easy; last week a woman I was helping let go and fell on top of me".

At some stage, while exploring far north Queensland, I had decided to go to NZ for a holiday with Jeff. Somehow by then we had become more than travel buddies, deciding that planning a life together into the next phase was a good idea. Uncharted territory for us both, yet simply made sense.

Our families were curious. They saw our happiness through the occasional social media postings. There was to be no grand announcement or status update. We were happy to keep living, and camping and planning together.

Then NZ's open border with Australia closed. For the second time in fifteen months, I was not allowed to go to NZ. There would be no holiday. Jeff's plans to see his daughter on her birthday were not possible. Even getting back to South Australia or Victoria seemed impossible.

The day we were to fly home to NZ, we watched Jeff's uncle's funeral streamed from Taranaki, New Zealand. We sat on a hill in Brisbane, unaware that the city was heading into lockdown as well.

By the time the funeral finished, the Premier had declared that by 3 pm, Brisbane would lock down. We had to act fast. We escaped inland, keeping our distance from the public by finding isolated campsites, licking our wounds at not being able to travel to NZ and planning our next move. We would take a detour of about 3000 km. As a bonus, I got to see Muttaburrasaurus, a dinosaur whose remains were discovered by Doug Langdon near Muttaburra in 1963, and stayed in a town called Boulia, the home of the min min lights, a supernatural phenomenon. Both legends with stories as long as the roads leading to them. Along with a crew of scaffolders who were all Maori, we watched the All Blacks play in a bar called 'cuzzie bro' in Barcaldine. Here I stood under the tree of knowledge, learned of the Shearers Strike in 1891, and the beginning of the Labour Party of Australia.

There was a census. Jeff and I filled out our forms and registered our coordinates of where our tent was that night. We were counted.

With so much uncertainty again mounting with coronavirus restrictions, we both knew we needed to get work. I hadn't finished being a midwife in Australia after all. The new concept of being a couple changed the employment stakes. Where I preferred to work, there would be no sheep to shear. Where the good shearing was, midwifery didn't appeal.

We learned the art of compromise. Neither had needed to do this for many years. We hoped it would be worth it.

As it happened, I got a job in Swan Hill and Jeff would rather reluctantly return to Victoria to shear sheep.

Travelling during coronavirus across borders again held little excitement. It had become burdensome and we were aware of the need to avoid NSW who were getting record numbers of coronavirus cases. Australia was colour coding the pandemic. My well-practised expertise in border pass applications finally failed. I was perplexed. As we had been in a red zone and South Australia was in an orange zone, the bureaucrats were still making the rules up as they went. Trying to get two people across the border, Jeff with a SA residential address and me with a permit to travel, was too much for me.

"Let's just wait and see if there is any border patrol for SA," I said.

As we drove the unsealed, uninhabited Birdsville track, I thought about a lovely nurse who was in the flat next door to me in the accommodation at Tennant Creek. One afternoon around the pool, We were talking about midwifery and premie babies. She told me her story. "I was one of them. I arrived a bit early. From what they tell me it was a hurry up cause she's probably going to die so name her and baptise her. So they did. Dr G apparently said to my parents, "where there's life, there's hope.

"And so mum and dad chose my middle name as Marree because it's the start of a long hard track. Dad worked out there on stations so he knows a rough hard track. But poor mum didn't get any care I don't think because they thought she was the Aunty because she was up walking around she told me. They didn't know what to do with babies like that. Pretty happy with my name because people who loved me gave that to me even considering what some people said to them they still hoped for the best."

"How early were you born?" I asked.

"24 weeks. Back in rural NSW though they knew fuck all. Ma's doctor didn't even come to see her when she said she went into labour. They got the helicopter to fly me to Brisbane. She's still annoyed that they took 7 hrs to fly when they said if she survives for five hours we'll take her."

What a story. I said to Jackie, "but you're not that old, so it wasn't that long ago?"

"No but I have a big scar on my belly. Some nurse apparently tore off the Elastoplast that was tying down the tubes. They weren't used to looking after ones like that and had no special unit and all that. I'm alright though. I'm more than lucky."

When Jackie Marree told me this story, I hadn't heard of either the Birdsville Track nor Marree, and to be honest never thought I'd ever be driving it. But here we were. Coming from the north, Marree was at the end of a long hard track alright.

The Birdsville track traverses three deserts along its route, the Strzelecki Desert, Sturt Stony Desert and Tirari Desert. As we drove, I thought the reaction to the whole pandemic seemed distorted

"It all seems so stupid," I said to Jeff. "Coronavirus would never survive in these deserts."

Marree came into view as a watering hole in the distance. A sprinkle of buildings heralding the tracks end and habitation. It was here we were almost stymied by another border patrol.

"Shit. I hope they don't make us go back up the track," I said to Jeff as the officer put his sun hat on and came over to our car.

"Good afternoon," said the tall middle-aged policeman. His offsider remained in his vehicle, reading a novel.

"Hello," said Jeff. "Hi," I said, smiling.

"Have you got your official blah blah blah South Australian pass?" he asked. Every state in Australia had their own app and its own pass acronym. We were now going to be crossing our 4th border in less than three months.

"I have my V Pass," I said, secretly knowing that it would not be enough, but deciding to play the dumb tourist and hoping to get away with it. "I start work next week in Swan Hill."

"Swan Hill, Victoria?" he asks.

"So, how are you going to get there?"

"We are avoiding NSW like the plague," Jeff waits for the policeman to get his joke,

He didn't blink an eyelid. "We will go through Narrocourt," Jeff continued.

"Have you got your blah blah blah official south Australian pass, though?" he asks again.

"Oh, I didn't know we needed it," I lied. It was too difficult to say I knew we needed it, but I couldn't figure out how to use your stupid system, and your call centre workers didn't know either, so I gave up.

I added, "When I came through SA last year to go to Alice

Springs to work, I was allowed thirty-six hours to transit, so I thought it would be the same."

"Gosh, I'm so sorry." I lied. I almost heard a cock crow.

He was a good cop. We told him where we had been since the Brisbane three-day snap lockdown, where we were going to be in SA, explaining it was just to collect shearing gear and when we planned to be in Victoria.

"I'll see how I can help." He went back to his colleague, who got an iPad out and tapped away.

He strolled back to our vehicle like a cowboy walking down the main street in a western movie. All the attention was on him and he knew we were going nowhere until he said so.

"So Teresa, you have 48 hrs in SA transit, and Jeff, you have to go back to your address and isolate there for fourteen days."

That's officially what I'm telling you to do. Understand?

We both nodded and thanked him for helping us out.

The town where Jeff had his tools was two days driving to even get there. That address was a flat he no longer lived in, and his kit was in a garage locked up. We felt like refugees. Arriving in SA we knew the temperatures would plummet, so we booked into a cabin, overstayed our 48 hrs and left as soon as practicable to Victoria, only 30km across the border. Tantalisingly close.

That morning I was like, " How come we can just drive into Victoria?" There are no border patrols or anything. Bloody stupid coronavirus rules. I went on a rant. There was so much unnecessary stress. I just wanted to get to Swan Hill and start work. Everywhere was desperate for midwives and sheep shearers.

I was mid-rant when we passed a police vehicle that did a u-turn and flashed its lights.

"God, what now?" Jeff said

The South Australia number plates in Victoria alerted the policeman.

Jeff showed his Victoria entry permit, and the officer didn't even acknowledge me.

Too hard," I thought. Too right mate, I'm over it and best you don't even ask me.

I'm glad thought bubbles are silent.

Jeff drove off. I'm always amazed at how calm he remains.

"Well, we are here in Victoria," he said. "Where will we stay?" Realising that we hadn't actually planned the next leg of our journey, we both looked at the dark clouds and said at the same time

"Motel."

Although it was not a humorous situation, we started laughing. It would all be all right.

I emailed Swan Hill via my agency to ask if Jeff could stay with me at my accommodation for the weekend. We hadn't even thought of where Jeff would actually work let alone live. I would go to the hospital, meet the midwifery ward crew, and settle into the digs. I didn't have a car, so Jeff would sort out groceries etc.

But the managers at Swan Hill replied with a curt, bordering on rude reply, essentially saying no to Jeff, but reluctantly allowing him two nights due to exceptional circumstances. They would charge him $100 a night.

"Welcome to Swan Hill," I thought. "Bugger them, let's stay here in the Grampians, and I'll turn up on Monday, and they will have to show me my room during work time."

As if we had not had enough running from Coronavirus lockdowns, the whole state of Victoria went into another lockdown that weekend. With short notice Dan, the man, their Premiere, made the very unpopular announcement.

I was beginning to feel like I knew every state Premiere and more about Australian politics than most Australians, and certainly, more than I actually wanted to know.

So here we were in a motel in the Grampian national park on a Saturday morning; it was freezing cold - relatively so - as we had just spent three months in the desert. I had single accommodation from Monday and a job. Jeff had no job and nowhere to live. Caravan parks were mostly closed. It was hard to remain optimistic.

So we went for a steep exhausting walk and tired ourselves out of overthinking. Taking in the views of green-covered mountains and steep valleys diverted our attention. We had been so very lucky to avoid Coronavirus; we had not been locked in our house in a city. As my children continued to remind me, we still had freedom. This was just a hiccup. It would all sort out.

The kind and accommodating motel owner kept our room available in case Jeff couldn't get accommodation in Swan Hill. As it happened, the caravan park owner, who was anti-government, had room for Jeff. I was shown my accommodation, we both stocked up with supplies and for the first night in three months, we slept in different houses. It was surprisingly empty.

Monday morning first day at Swan Hill.

The staff were pleasant, and as the newbie agency midwife, I was welcomed and given a brief rundown of where everything was, shown the roster and put to work. Jeff busied himself with some vehicle maintenance and personal admin. Our lives had taken on a completely different trajectory than both had imagined. Ten weeks ago, we were friends embarking on a road trip. We were going to be parting ways in Brisbane. Jeff was to be in NSW shearing, and I was going to be in London. But here we were in Swan Hill, I having come full circle back to Victoria and Jeff in a state he didn't really want to be in. We had become an item. So much had changed. We both needed time to readjust.

My first week was a mixture of shifts and meeting people. Jeff came to my accommodation for meals, and he had shearing contractors to call. On my first day off, we went for a walk around a lake a few kilometres out of Swan Hill.

As we were chatting about how lovely this area was, I fell. Not just a simple fall but a great ankle rolling trip on the part of the new tarmac path that had sunken into a huge divet[3]. I must have gathered momentum as when my wrist met the ground, I felt and heard the smashing, and the pain was instant even with the outpouring of adrenalin.

My career, my accomodation and my income seemed to vanish in that instance. And I was in Australia and couldn't get home. Neither to London nor New Zealand. It was a dark hour.

So within a week, I had gone from one side of the bed to sitting in ED on the other. And what an insight that was to be. I'm a midwife but am also a nurse, it wasn't rocket science to know that I had fractured something. Three nurses came and took obs, gave me name tags, and asked questions. Not one introduced themselves or asked how I was. I was in such pain and shock. I was alone as coronavirus rules dictated "no family."

The radiologist was so very kind. I had actually met him the day before, so said to him, I'm sure I'm just imagining I have broken something, as I looked at the limp disfigured angle of my hand. He unofficially let me know that I had a comminuted fracture of the distal radius and possible fractured ulna. I knew the pain was real.

The locum anaesthetist was not only a good-looking young man but also kind, efficient, and had a professional and positive bedside manner. He and the on-call recovery nurse provided excellent care as I was wheeled away into the theatre for stabilising.

That was when the good care finished.

"You can go home now," said my allocated nurse, who had not introduced herself. "Where are your clothes?"

I was awake but sleepy from the light anaesthetic. "Um, I don't know?" I have a bright blue top somewhere," I said.

"Where did you take it off?"

I had been in ED triage, radiology, Pre-op, OT and now back in the ED corridor. I had no recollection.

The nurse was annoyed as she pulled the curtain after her and left.

"Ta da," she said as she bounced through the curtain, presenting my top. "I found it."

You are not a bloody miracle worker, I thought, but did not say.

"Thanks, that's it," I said instead.

With that, she left again.

"Do I have any pain medication to take home?" I asked a nurse who poked her head in the curtain.

"Oh, I'm not looking after you; I was just seeing if Dalia was in here," she said

So that was her name?

Dalia returned.

"Can I have some pain relief to take home?"

"You have had a lot in theatre. Pick some ibuprofen up at the supermarket," she said. She smiled and left.

I felt horrible. I felt ashamed that I was part of this profession.

I got off the bed and struggled with getting dressed. I couldn't get my arm through my bright blue top, so I just pulled one arm through and the top down, covering my hand that was in a back slab. The top only barely covered my back.

My shoes had been placed in a hospital property bag with my phone.

I texted Jeff. Come and get me NOW.

There was no way I could manage to get the laces of my boots undone for me to put my feet in, so I just put the phone in one shoe and carried them.

Dalia came back as I was about to leave.

"Haven't you got any shoes?" she asked.

"I can't manage to get them on," I confessed, holding back my tears, expecting her to come to my rescue.

"Oh," she shrugged, then left.

So I walked out of the ED at Swan Hill hospital, a staff member, bawling my eyes out and barefooted.

When Jeff arrived, I couldn't even talk.

He moved into my room with me and became my carer, my cook, and my companion.

When the managers heard of my accident, they were so supportive and surprisingly allowed me to stay on for free at the accommodation that was provided. This was possibly the kindest thing an organisation had done during my accidental time in

Australia. I had heard of agency nurses getting sick and being kicked out of their accommodation the next day. I had eight weeks of recovery, and further surgery to stabilise the fracture with pins and plate. This went a long way to compensate for the abysmal nursing care I had received in ED. I never told anyone about my experience until I left.

41 NEW ZEALAND'S BIGGEST LOTTERY

Diary entry: from Swan Hill

It's almost two years since I left London, and today, I entered the lottery for a third time in my attempt to secure a room in managed isolation so I can go home to New Zealand.

My attempt was unsuccessful. My creative writing group in Highgate will meet face to face for the first time in eighteen months. I will join them via zoom. For my homework, I've submitted this reflective essay.

I feel as welcome as a nuclear submarine.

A few years back, I left New Zealand to start a new life.

So what? Isn't that what many New Zealanders do?

My forebears left Ireland knowing they would not return; however, I left New Zealand knowing I would. I'm a traveller. It is in my blood.

A proud Kiwi, I have a strong southland accent and, like most Kiwis abroad, act unwittingly as ambassadors for Aotearoa, New Zealand every day.

London has been my home for the last decade.

In 2019, as the RWC final was underway in Japan, I landed in Melbourne for six months of sunshine and to spend time with my newlywed son and his wife.

Plans to return to London via New Zealand were stymied by the drama that was unfolding out of China. On the 20th of March 2020, the curtains were pulled across the Tasman, and I became a displaced person, a fugitive maybe or simply a covid refugee.

I'm still here.

From relatively virus-free, sunshine-filled Australia, I watched in horror as Europe shut down, daily statistics of cases, ventilators and deaths flooded the news channels. Two of my children were amid the EU/UK crisis. Friends succumbed to the virus, long Covid was a thing. I worried, willing all to stay safe mentally and physically. My youngest son lived alone in London, minding my rented flat. He started a new job working from home and for the first year never met his colleagues, remaining socially isolated for months on end.

My second daughter graduated from Cambridge University, UK, got engaged, built a new home, and planned her wedding in my absence.

My Melbourne Whānau endured the first two lockdowns, threw their savings into paying rent with no income to fill the coffers, pulled the pin on their Australian dream and are now establishing a new life in Latvia.

My eldest daughter was grateful she had returned to Wellington, New Zealand from her Nordic holiday just before being caught in a foreign land, is cocooned safely in the Covid free bubble: for now, anyway.

The Antipodes had the edge in the early days. Open space and the ability to close borders. But SARS-Cov-2 arrived, predictably in my mind, eventually. We all knew it couldn't be detained at the NZ border. Those of us on the outside knew. Many on the inside still deny this reality.

I've tried to remain optimistic. My microbiology background gives me an educated appreciation of viruses, mutations, and vaccinations. It won't be easy. It won't be quick.

I'm frequently told I'm lucky to be in Australia. I pretend I am.

Two years on, my London life has been packed up, business placed in hibernation as I remain holed up in Australia.

I'm here. I'm here by accident. I've written this book about my time working rural and remote indigenous communities, keeping positive, thinking it would be over by now. The last chapter has been written many times. It seems there will be more.

Meanwhile, Covid endures and lives up to the reputation as causing a Global Pandemic.

My views are out of synch with many Kiwis, and I've been unfriended by my oldest nursing buddy, accused of wanting to spread the virus by Whānau, invitations to stay revoked by friends and vitriolic replies to social media posts from a Teacher in Cromwell! I never did like teachers.

We all have a Covid story. I'm in good company. There are over 30,000 expat Kiwis who want to go home and like me, can't. Aotearoa New Zealand is still playing the game of keeping Covid out. They won't win. Sadly, the fringe theorists are fuelling paranoia and fear. The previously kind and welcome arms of New Zealand are as though thalidomide has been consumed.

I want to go home. I can't pretend I'm lucky anymore.

Australia has announced a deal with the UK and America to build a nuclear-powered submarine. This will inflate the already fractured relations with China. France has been kicked in the goolies. A broken contract.

"We have not and will not ever accept nuclear powered submarines in New Zealand waters," Aunty Jacinda says.

I protested for a nuclear free New Zealand.

Today I'm Number 22791 in the queue of the revamped MIQ system where we are playing the game of 'who gets a Quarantine Bed in a stinky Hotel'.

I'm not going to inoculate Aotearoa with the virus of the century.

Apart from being fully vaccinated, I haven't a hope of getting into MIQ.

I feel as welcome as a nuclear submarine.

Perhaps I'll take a lotto ticket- maybe those numbers are more likely to come up.

Two weeks ago, I fell over and felt the crush of a fracture in my wrist. What flashed before me was not that I was going to be unable to work and my career may be over, it was the knowing that I could not go home.

All fingers are pointing at me and thirty thousand others from under the curtains.

You left, you had plenty of opportunities to return, why do you think you are so special, we stayed and paid tax, house prices are up because of you.

The blinds are still drawn.

Along with my bones, my wairua[4] was fractured that day.

I now sport nine pins and two plates under the new plastic alternative to plaster of Paris.

The only certainty I know is at least my wrist will mend.

42 THAT FEELING A MIDWIFE GETS

It's a hard thing to describe, but it was after I returned to work that I had a sense of doom.

Logically, I accepted that I was stressed about my future; plans had drastically changed. I had come out to Australia for six months of sunshine and was to return to my former life with enthusiasm and energy to grow my business.

The monthly storage bill reminded me I still have belongings in London. The annual mooring fees for my narrow boat seem to have come around all too quickly, and when I saw a Suzuki Vitara here in Ozzie, I had a moment of sadness. It really was a good vehicle. I still feel awful about my daughter Hannah's 'stuff' that was left in the boot. I didn't know that when the scrap man took it away.

Australia had surprised me with its beauty, and apart from the heat, spiders flies, and snakes, and don't forget the frogs, it was a place I was learning to love. That surprised me because I feel as though I've been resisting Australia, keeping her at arm's length, only being here by accident.

My life buddy and I oscillate between where to live: NZ, OZ, London, or Ireland.

This gut feeling or sense of doom was likely because of my situation. It wasn't logical, yet I just couldn't shake it.

I had been in nursing and midwifery for forty years and had not had any unexpected bad outcomes. My worst fear was that a mother or baby would die on my shift. My fear was quite specific. I couldn't shake it, and it annoyed me because I knew about the power of thought. I found myself reluctant to change shifts – this could be tempting fate.

I suspected it was anxiety. I'd never experienced it before. It wasn't healthy, so I tackled it head-on and said affirmations and positive statements each day as I went to work.

Then my doom premonition was realised.

A new obstetrician had just started at midday. She had never locumed at Swan Hill but was an experienced consultant. It was Monday and busier than usual as the hospital had been on bypass since Thursday. Bypass means the women have to go to another hospital as it is deemed unsafe for a birth due to staff shortage. Our permanent obstetrician had contracted coronavirus. In December, the bypass had been because of midwifery shortages.

A thirty-eight week pregnant woman had come in for review. She was unknown to our service, had had little antenatal care, and had been treated for hypertension but had not taken her medication. This was her 4th baby. She was on a CTG foetal monitor as part of her obstetric assessment.

A sixteen-year-old who had started with a triplet pregnancy but was now carrying twins, was in the birthing room also on a CTG. She was in a hurry to leave as sixteen-year-olds are.

One midwife had called in sick, and the afternoon midwife had arrived.

Two new mums had come in for baby weight and wellbeing checks. The obstetrician was seeing another outpatient for review of a rash, and the midwife antenatal clinic was running.

By 4 pm, my colleague from the morning shift was still busy. Her thirty eight week pregnant mum with hypertension needed to be transferred to Bendigo, so she needed to stay to complete the process.

Meanwhile, Kayley, second-time mum scheduled for induction on the day the hospital went on bypass and had been rebooked, arrived with bags packed and ready to have her baby.

I went to Kayley to explain there would be a delay and found she was anxious and had built anxiety over the days when the hospital was on bypass. So, I sat and just chatted. We had lots in common as it turned out. She was from Dublin and lived in Mataura, a small town in NZ close to my hometown. She worked as a roustabout for years, so we had a good laugh about life in the shearing sheds.

Then midwife H came into the room. "Teresa, I need your help. We have a Cat 1 section."

The woman was in the small birthing room. The CTG was on, and fetal bradycardia, dangerously low heart rate was evident. I turned the mum onto her left lateral and repositioned the monitor. I introduced myself and asked her name.

Nakita was an older woman. Her face had the lines of a smoker and an Ozzie tan. She looked me in the eye and asked, "Jimmy, will I call Jimmy?"

"Yes, tell him you are going to have your baby."

"Can he come in?" "Yes, of course he can; tell him to come to the maternity ward."

I knew the baby would be out before he arrived. He had been sent home to get Nakita's belongings for her to take to Bendigo.

She phoned him. Her voice was crackly.

We attended the practical disrobing of the bottom half of her clothing, grabbed the catheterisation equipment, and wheeled her in to the OT.

I threw on some scrubs, hat and boot cover as OT staff prepared her. I realised I had never been into the OT at this hospital. They all look the same, but different.

The theatre staff were preparing Nakita on the operating table. It was busy. We took the baby monitor off, and I popped the catheter in. Theatre staff are always so happy to see a midwife for this task.

The room was filled with staff. The junior midwife who had been caring for her had scrubbed to accept the baby. The doctors were waiting by the resuscitare[5], after checking it.

I knew only two of the staff. I felt so sorry for the obstetrician and remembered that I had asked her if she knew where the OT was. We had joked that she hoped she wouldn't need it but knew she would be pointed in the right direction.

Here we all were. My first time in SH theatre. A locum obstetrician who had only started four hours ago. And a pregnant mother who we had very little knowledge about.

My thoughts were now for the baby, so I stayed as support, although there were already two midwives and two doctors waiting.

The baby was out and cried. What a relief!

I thought, it's time I left as I was not needed.

But the focus changed to the woman. The raised voice drew our attention. "Start CPR," he said.

"This is it, I thought- this is what I knew was going to happen." the woman had gone into cardiac arrest.

A nurse started chest compressions. Although I was well out of the way, I took a step backwards and grounded myself by putting my hands on the wall. I would not need to be part of the resus. I stared. I was in shock.

I watched the chest bouncing down down down. I had never been in an arrest situation involving an obstetric client.

Another staff member ran out, "I'm calling code blue," and within two seconds, I heard, "Code blue OPERATING THEATRE' CODE BLUE OPERATING THEATRE."

"Have you got Adrenalin?" said the loud voice.

"Adrenalin given," someone replied.

Another person ran to get a step for the person doing chest compressions.

Changeover was the order.

Press, press, press, I felt that my eyes were wide open, watching with intrigue how deep the chest was compressed, how bendy it was.

The defibrillator arrived.

"Stand back," said the loud voice.

Everyone stared at the cardiac monitor.

"Well done. Well done," said the loud voice.

No defibrillation needed.

Professionally cool as cucumbers, the surgery continued.

I looked at the wee baby girl on the recussitaire who was alert and pink. She would probably never know her mother's heart had stopped beating just as she took her first breath.

I was stunned. It was my cue to leave.

Back on the ward, I popped in to see Kayley and reassure her as much as anything, as she would have heard the code blue.

In the nursery, Midwife K, a retired but experienced midwife who had been on call, was wrapping the baby.

Dad arrived, shocked and disorientated.

"What is it?" he asked.

I said, "Here, come and have a look for yourself."

Midwife K was grumpy and said, "It's a girl." What a shame, I thought. She needn't have been so officious, and this new father was denied the second of gender revelation.

He then said, "What about mum?"

"Oh, she is doing fine, here, have a hold of this wee one," I said. I hoped I was telling the truth.

The tall, burly man was crying as he sat holding his firstborn in his arms.

The vision of the baby's mum's chest being compressed was stuck in my mind.

"Congratulations," I said. "Isn't she just so beautiful?"

At that moment, I remembered there was no baby milk on the ward. It had been ordered but hadn't arrived. I had given an extra couple of bottles to the mum who had gone home on Wednesday and used the last one for a mum who had come into the ward for a domiciliary check the day before.

Now was not the time to insist on putting this wee baby to the breast. Her mum would be closely monitored for a few hours at least.

I headed out to the supermarket and bought a tin of baby formula.

The baby was going to be transferred to Bendigo. Nakita was stable.

When I got home, I was still in shock. I did, however, have a sense of calm as well.

The feeling of doom had gone.

I had a large glass of NZ Reisling. Tomorrow is another day, as we say.

I had been invited to the code blue debrief via Zoom the following day.

This was a non-event. Everyone was given a chance to say what went well, and what went not so well (can't say what went wrong, apparently).

The theatre staff patted themselves on the back for having successfully resuscitated the woman. They had indeed worked well and saved her life.

My impression was that the Anaesthetist was just relieved the woman was alive, as was the Obstetrician. Neither had this ever happened to a pregnant/ intrapartum woman. That was a club I too was in.

I suggested that it could have been very handy if, amidst the sea of blue scrubs and masks that, we could have name tags and role definitions that identify the staff. This is a work in progress, but I hear it is being initiated.

What wasn't said was loud. I hope for another forum to investigate what actually went wrong for this woman.

A cascade of events from a woman who took little responsibility for her own health, presenting with underlying medical problems predating her pregnancy. Lack of documented, easily accessible patient histories, lack of passing on relevant information to key stakeholders...the list goes on.

The mother and baby were separated for three days, the baby was being sent to a tertiary hospital for stabilising of sugars and temperature, the mother in HDU for stabilising her medical condition.

It was for all, staff included, a happy reunion when baby was back in her mother's arms. Both are doing well. For now.

43 THE JOURNEY CONTINUES

It seems unbelievable that I am still applying for a spot in New Zealand to quarantine in. This is my 8th attempt. Maria my colleague from Alice Springs days has returned for another contract and is on day 10 of her 14 days. It seems a hazy recollection of my early days of the pandemic. Quarantine, hundy club, my children all managing in different countries. My London life was on hold, now it had been packed neatly away. Lockdowns across Europe were continuing.

The world had pooled its resources with energy and optimism. The world was changing day by day. It was hard to imagine a new normal. For now Jeff and I had to make the most of what we had infront of us. No one knew the ending.

The irony was that I was homesick. And I didn't even know where home was any more.

44 RESIGNATION AGAIN

Still stuck in Australia. Not all work though.

I had happily worked the remainder of my contract in Swan Hill. My Kiwi colleague who was an anti-vaxer had her contract revoked because she refused to "get the jab." She got a MIQ room. NZ is welcome to her, I secretly thought. The irony was that of two midwives applying for a spot, the one who can't work in NZ and refuses to be immunised, gets to go home.

Jeff and I had settled into an easy lifestyle making the most of our time in Victoria and 'going with the flow' regarding future plans, which were dependent on the NZ borders. I had joined the Facebook group 'grounded Kiwis' who were an amazing support to the thousands of us who could not return home. My situation was insignificant compared to many who had lost jobs, homes, and family members, and had babies alone, that list went on. It was tragic on so many levels. But week after week, we would all log on to the MIQ website at whatever hour it happened to be and try again again and again.

Jeff had been working with a contractor from a town fifty kilometres from Swan Hill, called Kerang. He had been offered the use of a cottage on one of the roustabout's parents' farm. Sarah Jane had been talking with Jeff, and when she found out he was living in one of the contractor's rooms, she was horrified. He had a reputation for being pretty rough around the edges. She arranged for both of us to see the cottage and could rent it if we liked.

And we did like it. We became firm friends of the family, sharing shearing stories, and local knowledge, and I was delighted to introduce Glenice to Prosecco, which was partaken of every Friday night. Dennis stuck with the beer.

I was asked to extend my contract and was happy to do so, but I had a holiday booked over Christmas and New Year. Jeff and I spent two weeks back in the trusty Toyota with our tent and were both in our happy place.

45 REMINDERS THAT I AM A MIDWIFE

With all that was happening in my world, I started to feel disconnected from who I was. We had a fabulous time in our wee tent meeting fascinating people, like the ex-prison officer who had a wine cellar of over 4000 bottles of red wine, all bought from the Barossa Valley, Montepulciano d'Abruzzo, or Spain. He lived on a farm, and had wall-to-ceiling collector books, one of which had Henry VIII's signature (a copy of the original of which there were only 300 worldwide).

And there was the old couple at Lakes Entrance. We had been driving for some hours, and my back was a little stiff. A walk along the seafront would fix it. I was enjoying the warmer weather and loving the freedom of simple clothing and jandals as we set off paddling into the contrasting cold sea and hot yellow sand. I found myself daydreaming of the simple things in life that bring pleasure, and laughing at my slowness at noticing the rogue waves that inevitably would rise up the legs of my shorts until even my knickers were wet. Not that I was bothered. It would soon dry out, and wearing dark shorts meant that it did not look like I had pee'd myself. The town we had stopped in had the curious name of Lakes

Entrance, and it became clear that the name was aptly named after a man-made shipway from the ocean to lakes. The entrance was called the narrows and consisted of large concrete blocks whitewashed that heralded the entrance. Lining each side were huge boulders, stacked one upon the other in a way that rough waves would not bother, sloping down to a base of rocks where crustaceans blackened them, and crabs, once spotted made the boulders shimmer with movement. The deep blue rolling waves nudged and crashed away in comfortable synergy. I watched a solo boat line up in the centre of the narrows and ride the waves and purge its engine to safely navigate into the calm lake. As I leaned on the rails, cooled by the sea breeze and mesmerised by the coming and goings of the waves and the boat, I caught my first glimpse of a dolphin fin. I called and pointed like a child; being the first to spot the dolphins is always a sense of one-upmanship - not quite a Livingston moment but a small feel-good factor as if I had planned their appearance. Good news travels fast, and the calmer water inside the entrance soon filled with kayakers, jet skis and fishing boats. I felt like they were intruding and disrupting the dolphin play time. Maybe they were used to it? I headed along the boardwalk quietly, pleased the sea mammals, which now included seals, had stopped playing - the boaties lost interest.

There was a frail elderly man stooped with age, balancing against the rail. His heavy black looking binoculars seemed to almost cause him to topple. He was looking back towards the narrows.

"Did you see the dolphin?" I asked as a way of greeting.

He slowly lowered the binoculars. I could see by his sun-weathered skin that he was well used to the outdoors. "Ive just spotted a seal but I don't know if it's alive," he replied.

"See that one down on the rocks? It floated right past me, and it was hard to tell if he was ok or not. Here have a look." He handed me the binoculars. I almost had to brace myself to hold them. I turned the smooth lenses to my focus, and the clarity of the view was amazing.

"Oh, I see what you mean," I said. "Let's hope he is just sleeping? I think they do that, don't they?"

"He chuckled "I don't know, really - he looked crook to me."

I called to Jeff and passed the eyepiece to him. "Can you see the seal? Have a look and see if you think he is dead or not?" Jeff handed the old man his binoculars and said, "I will go and check him out," and strode off down to the rocks.

"I've been watching those two dolphins out there actually - can you see them?" The old man looked to where I was pointing, and we waited for the brown form to surface upon a wave which it soon did.

"Oh yes, they look ok. That's good," he said. We stood watching the wildlife now uninhibited by any boats or canoeist who had left to explore the lakes.

"The dolphins will be back soon," the man said with a kind and intelligent tone as he returned to the bench to help himself to a sandwich. I hadn't been aware of the other person sitting on the bench until then. From a distance I was not quite sure if she was a man or a woman as age sometimes does move the prettiness of youth into the wisdom of wrinkles. She was elderly too; she smiled and I was welcomed with worn yellow teeth, bright blue eyes, and wispy hair. She wore a paisley long-sleeved shirt and taupe pants. The hat completed the Australian outback look.

"Hello," I said, "This is an amazing spot isn't it?" "Yes," she replied. Her voice was strong but gentle. "I'm afraid we have been spoilt here - the first time we came, we had a whole pod of dolphins swimming up and down right there, and she pointed to where her husband had been standing. It is a hard act to follow, but I hope you will see a dolphin soon."

I was curious or maybe, to be honest, nosey, and envious. What an amazing couple. A fair age, hitting eighty something and still out and about enjoying life.

"Where are you from?" she asked.

The man was balancing an egg topping on his bread, and he made his way to Jeff, who had returned from his "Is the seal dead or alive venture." I sat on the seat beside the lady and said, "I'm a Kiwi but lived in London until coronavirus."

Oh, she said and with a big smile. "I'm actually from England - do you know Croydon?"

"Yes, I do know Croydon. My friend Emma has just left Croydon to emigrate to NZ - so it's still happening.

"Oh well, I'm sure Croydon is different now. I left in 1954."

"Oh, were you a ten-pound pom then?"

She smiled and said, "Yes. Croydon was more or less a small town back then, but when I went back eighteen or so years ago, it was hardly recognisable. Bill and I live in Bendigo now. We retired there but come to the sea as often as we can."

"Oh, I was in Bendigo last week. We went to Hanging Rock but were too scared to take a picnic."

She laughed.

Bill and Jeff were deep in discussion about the seal. Jeff said it was hard to tell if he was just sleeping or not.

The lady had lovely posture, and her body language projected interest. She asked "What keeps you in London?"

I'm a midwife, but it's more that I love to travel across Europe that keeps me there. It certainly isn't the weather".

The easy conversation continued as we both shared parts of our life stories – both, I felt, were as interested in each other's. Having babies inevitably came up when I spoke about the hospital I had worked in.

"My first son was born in Canada," the woman said. "Bill was a civil engineer and we lived there for four years. It was horrible," she continued.

"Epidurals were new then, and they insisted that I have one. Terrible things," she said. "Is this your experience?"

I wasn't sure if she was asking professionally or personally. " Gosh," I replied "I didn't know epidurals were around back then. I knew in NZ they were available in the bigger cities in the late 70s, but the 50's, well, I'm really surprised." I spoke for a while about trends in birthing that are now prominent.

She smiled, "My second baby was born prematurely on the banks of the river in Heidleburgh, Germany. My waters broke and I said to Bill, this is it! They were very good to me there. She was 6lb, and the doctor put me up in his apartment, part of their house. I sent Bill back to the UK to get a job, and a house and the doctor gave me a big square pillow to carry my baby in. At the airport, the customs man asked what I had in the pillow. I said 'a baby girl.' They didn't believe me, and they didn't check. We just went through."

We both laughed, and I asked, "How does your daughter feel about being smuggled out of Germany on a pillow?" "She has been back and went to the hospital, where she was looked after. It is always good to go back to your roots - don't you agree?" I did and said it is really important.

"My next baby was born at home - the UK is all geared up for a home birth. Bill worked on the M3. He designed the road train." The woman seemed to be proud of this and explained how the road train was a train that went along tracks laying a concrete base for the road, smoothing and pressing as it went. When we went back, the road still had the same foundation. "That is impressive," I said. "A good thing for Bill to put on his CV," she laughed. "At eighty odd I don't think we need a CV." We both giggled a little. Wow, eighty odd - no wonder her teeth were worn - I had noticed Bill's false plate rattled in his mouth as he spoke, but she still had her own.

"We went back to where Bill worked in Kent, Devon - quite near Canterbury actually," she said.

I was thinking how very interesting her birth stories were when she said, "Then we emigrated to Australia and I had to have my son in a hospital. I told them I wanted to have my baby at home, but Australia didn't have the facilities for emergency blood like the UK. I really didn't want to go to the hospital but had no choice," she said.

Fascinating birth stories.

"So apart from raring four children, did you also have a career?

"When we knew we were emigrating, I got a job with the bank. The ANZ was part of the union bank in England so they said I could get a transfer. So that's what I did. I arrived in Sydney and walked into the newly independent ANZ bank where I met my first friend. She was sitting up on a high stool with all the cheques piled up. She had an ink pen and was ledgering the debits by hand. Then I was really lucky. As the new machines for ledger came in, I went around the branches teaching the staff how to use them. Young people these days have no idea how far the banking system has come. Of course, it is all automated now, but it wasn't that long ago; it was all done by hand."

"I really did love my job," she said. "But I saw an advertisement for an air hostess with TAA. I applied," she said "and realised I was too heavy. I weighed ten stone, so I changed how I ate and got to eight and half stone and became an air hostess. And I'm still eight and half stone. It served me well, didn't it Bill?" He gave an impartial nod.

"Sometime during my hostess days, we were at my girlfriend's house, and from behind the door, he peeped out. I ended up typing his masters' work. My dad was in the paper business, so we had it covered. I could type a bit. But he failed, so I had to leave him for a while so I didn't distract him. She was grinning and looking at her husband who was deep in conversation with Jeff, who had finished taking photos of the seals.

We said our goodbyes as I walked further along the path, contemplating how often being a midwife opens up conversations, and quite personal reflections. Her story was so insightful.

The sea was rough, and although the signs were explicitly warning us not to swim the canal, it was obviously not something I would ever entertain. Jeff was ahead, and I could see that something was distracting him in the water. Coming up to him, I, too, saw the slithery black form surfing the waves and diving for its food for the day. How lovely. More seals. So far, this Ozzie holiday had turned to be a veritable feast of flora and fauna. The road signs were everywhere on the walking tracks, the main highways and town entrances, either warning of the presence of venomous snakes or alerting the drivers to the possibility of a kangaroo bouncing onto the road. We had seen almost all of the native animals. The eastern brown snake was the least savoury on our remote walking track, but it was followed by kangaroo, koala, possum, kookaburra, and parakeet. And now seals in the wild were added and I had a faint hope that we might even see dolphins. Fingers crossed.

After listening to this amazing anecdote I found myself wondering if I still actually wanted to be a midwife. So much had changed. I was reflective, thinking back to before I had even arrived in Australia.

Our holiday continued. I felt like I was on a continuous holiday. It was a weird concept. We visited family and friends now that the NSW borders had opened and saw in the New Year of 2022, celebrating with my Aunt Be, my cousin and his partner. By now, our grounded Kiwi intel was whispering of NZ border changes, and so we made the bold decision to book our flights home for early March. We reconfirmed our place on the Milford Track Ultimate Hike and made vague plans to celebrate Jeff's 60th birthday along with an aunt's 50th wedding anniversary. We knew to keep plans fluid. I continued to apply for the MIQ spot. It was hopeless.

A few days further into our holiday, as we were returning to Swan Hill, I found myself reflecting on the early days of my time here, before I was here by accident. I had accepted a contract for five months in a Victorian town called Benalla. Getting a job from my flat in London was challenging, and I had started the application back in April when I had first decided to leave my London life for six months and indulge in the sunshine.

Now I have lost count of how many contracts I have taken on; different agencies have different systems, pay scales and attitudes to their health workers.

From my perspective, I've found agencies to be staffed by young and non-health experienced staff who are over-enthusiastic and promise you the world and haven't a clue what a midwife does for a job. I found myself impatient and would only give them one chance to sign me up. If they showed any signs that they neither knew what a midwife was, or they hadn't actually read my CV, I gave them the flick. A few got this. My best reply from one agency was, "Dear Teresa, I see by your application you do not feel competent in the delivery suite. I suggest you spend a couple of years updating your experience by working in delivery suites where you live, then get back in touch with us. We will be happy to find work for you in sunny Australia and are sure you would love to work here." I nearly lost my patience with that agency.

I had clearly stipulated I did not want to work in delivery suite, not that I was incompetent, yet I kept getting offers of jobs all over the country, all of which included labour and shift work. Even after clearly reiterating with one agent "only antenatal and postnatal positions and no night duty," I remember clearly driving up to sit outside the local high school at a very odd time of the early morning to interview for a position in Deniliquin. Phone reception in my flat could be inconsistent, hence the early morning drive. Ho hum, it was for the labour ward manager. Again the agency was focused on getting the commission for placement and really disinterested in the job specs. I apologised for wasting their time and gave the agency bimbo a bollocking telling her that I had got up in the middle of the night and did not appreciate being put forward for a position I would never want to take. And besides, the town sounds delinquent, so it would not work for me.

Two and a half years after that wasted phone interview, while accidentally in Australia, I drove through that wee town of Denelinqun or is it Delinquent, and was surprised how sweet a town it was, just along the Murray river from where I was living.

Leigh Dunn came to my rescue. LDH nursing recruitment. I don't know how I found her or she found me, but she listened, understood, and negotiated a contract for me in Benalla. Sure, I would be responsible for birthing women, but it was not a delivery suite, it was small, and there were GP obs who were happy to birth the babies and were available for emergencies. The annual birth rate in this town was under hundred, and I did catch a few babies while on shift.

I also registered with HCA, one of Australia's biggest agencies, and was able to secure a few metropolitan shifts in Melbourne when I went to the city to visit Ted and Liva. HCA was sophisticated and spot on for insisting on your competencies, providing online portals to keep up to date and in the days pre coronavirus (PC) in-house training sessions. Unfortunately, although HCA operates all over Australia, each state operates a different business, and so when applying to work rural and remote or in another state, many of the online learning is different, and this alone is time-consuming and tiresome. One thing I say to colleagues who ask me about working in Oz is that they must have the patience of a saint, and be prepared to do online training to wash hands and give out drugs. Be prepared to contact colleagues who may not remember you for your latest reference.

Coronavirus has so much to answer to. I sometimes reflect that if I had known I would still be in Australia two and a half years since I arrived and I would have done things differently. How different, I'm not sure, but maybe I would have gone to one of the places I loved to work, like Tennant Creek and bought myself a decent vehicle so I could explore the country. I would have enrolled in a Master's in something remotely interesting yet not to health orientated, and I would have engaged in the indigenous community, opened up my midwifery talents and made a good sum of money. Instead, I felt temporary and accidentally here, always thinking I would not be staying long, changing my mind about my future, trying to get to see my daughter in Wellington, pining for my kids in the northern hemisphere and feeling a little lost in the big continent of Australia.

Aotearoa closed the curtains to travellers, as I've already documented in March 2020. Then I couldn't get back to the UK either. Since then, although accidentally here, I found myself oscillating between going to NZ or going to UK but actually staying here.

NZ has been the most soul-destroying and frustrating coronavirus travesty I've encountered.

Each contract in Australia was for a few months, and I watched and waited, wondering what I should do. In April 2021, my son, who had sublet my flat in London, had had enough of living on his own, working on his own, and phoned me one day to say he needed to vacate the flat.

I totally understood his need to change something in his life. Coronavirus UK was horrid. Brexit UK was horrid.

So I had to let go of my flat, getting packers in to load up my small smattering of possessions and put them in storage. This itself was not a problem. Letting go of my former life was devastating. I'm not sure how or if I will ever recover from it. We all have a story. My casualty was my flat in Highgate, my Newborninthecity ™ business in London. My life in London was slowly being covidized. My friends were relocating back to NZ, and I realised the life I had left and planned to go back to, no longer existed.

Getting into NZ proved to be a nightmare, and I have over the months felt my Labour Party Whānau (forbears) turning in their graves. From my point of view, the reality that thousands of NZ citizens have had to beg and enter a lottery to return home is shameful. NZ, which I've represented to the rich and famous of Londons society and throughout Europe via kapahaka and Ngati Ranana, or simply through my work at the Portland hospital have slapped me in the face like the proverbial wet fish. Initially lauded as the best country to manage coronavirus, in my opinion, an "elimination policy" to keep coronavirus out at all costs has fostered a nation of paranoia, fear and mistrust. No longer the kind and open people, now the fear of coronavirus has left tens of thousands of her people alone, desperate, broke, and broken-hearted. While politicians', sports people, and entertainers can enter NZ easily, those whose loved ones are dying, whose families are separated, whose jobs have stopped sponsoring them in far-off countries, whose children are graduating, whose babies are being born without their dads, sisters are dying friends are crying are left to the lottery system of MIQ. Lest we ever forget how this Labour government has treated her citizens, I will not with a true heart be able to put a tick in that box at election time. I'm ashamed of the way the country is behaving. I detest how my family are reacting. I despise the entertainers for not standing up for those who cannot enter. It is a coronavirus shame. My uncle was the General Secretary for the Norman Kirk labour govt. I met Helen Clark and Jacinda Ardern, who was very pregnant, in London at the Topp Twins 60th Birthday party. I would never have ever thought that I would ever be banned from entering my birth country.

I phoned the help desk at the MIQ after my eighth attempt to secure a room to get into NZ. I spoke with a lovely Eastern European immigrant. He asked me, "Under what condition are you applying to return to NZ? I replied, "I was born in Bluff sixty years ago. My four children are eighth generation Pakeha, New Zealand. I'm very upset that I have to answer that question." He gently replied. "I can hear your distress in your voice, Teresa, I understand."

I think he actually did.

In the midst, I reconnected with a term called venting one's spleen. In doing so, I wrote a piece and sent it to the newspapers in NZ and to the very supportive Grounded Kiwis Facebook page. The spleen venting was nodded and commented upon, ticked and liked by the Facebook members, all of who were resonating with my sentiments. I never got any reply from the news hubs. Ho hum.

Meanwhile, Ozzie had snubbed the French, the diplomatic row over who would build the defence force submarines for their country was the hot topic and replaced the coronavirus data for a few hours, and the nuclear-powered submarines were the winners.

It is winter in Europe. Boris Johnson is being challenged for holding parties at number 10 during the strict UK lockdown last year while people died alone, and Queen Elizabeth was the only mourner at Prince Philip's funeral. My friends are back skiing in Austria, and holidaying in Spain and rapid antigen tests (RAT) are delivered to homes for screening. New Zealand is being accused of going from the revered managers of coronavirus to being the most backward. We have flights booked to Auckland in twenty nine day's time and have our vehicle and belongings to arrange to be sent. My tenants will need sixty one days' notice to vacate, and we await the NZ government's decision on the Omicron in the community as to whether the grounded Kiwis can return. The logistics are challenging. We are at the whim of the politicians. I wrote an email to Dr. Duncan Webb, the local politician I had voted for in the last election.

Dear Duncan,

I come from a long line of staunch Labour supporters, and my earliest memory of politics was as a child meeting Norman Kirk at my home when my uncle John Wybrow brought him around a meal. He was an inspirational gentleman and politician.

I have been living in Europe since 2003, and accidentally in Australia since Covid having voted for the labour candidate for Christchurch Central each election.

I am writing to advise you that I will NOT be voting for you nor any labour candidate in the next election and I will be voicing my dissent at any opportunity.

For all the years I have been living and working overseas I have been a New Zealand advocate and in my job, I met many high profile members of the public in London. With my strong Southland accent, the conversation easily turns to New Zealand.

I have toured Europe with London kapa haka rōpū and it was with incredible pride that I represented the most amazing country in the world.

My personal journey and story of failed MIQ applications is just one of many. I am not one of the thousands who are desperate to return due to family demise, personal health, financial hardship nor visa overstay status.

I am merely trying to return to NZ to live and set up my business.

I am currently in Australia going from town to town, contract to contract, living out of a suitcase now for over two years. My life in London has closed down due to Covid and I am one of many whose world has changed. I am trying to embrace the changes as a resilient Kiwi does.

However, the governments initial Covid response was as a choice an appropriate one, but from my perspective as a medical professional is now skewed . The citizens of Aotearoa are fuelled with propaganda and live in fear so much so that they cannot see what is happening around the world.

The "keep NZ safe" is out dated propaganda as the mental health of thousands and thousands of Kiwi is being threatened. This is purely because you have locked us out and locked many in.

A wall is by any other name still a wall. The MIQ is a wall.

Your government has prioritised rooms for sportsmen, businessmen, arts performers and cronies at the expense of her own citizens. Heaven forbid people have been able to come and go on holidays, get a spot for a friend's wedding, while others have watched parents die over Zoom, have been kicked out of countries, and relationships have ended due to not being allowed home to their country. Shame on you and your govt.

I have had eight failed MIQ applications.

I have had two failed relocation attempts (its not easy to leave a job and accommodation and be told you have to start again)

Shame on you for not stepping up for Kiwis abroad.

Shame on you and the govt for not being for the people.

Shame on you and the govt for locking thousands of Kiwis out of their country.

This is a black time for New Zealand.

Perhaps the grounded Kiwis court case, conveniently delayed by the judicial system will shine some legal light on the plight of citizens. Perhaps the pressure of Charlotte Bellis will finally help you and your govt to see how ridiculous you are all behaving perhaps the omicron will reach the magic numbers and home isolation will be available?

I am still hopeful to return in March. Logistics are challenging *and sadly the fear fuelled propaganda machine that I am covered in Covid and going to infect you all has split my family.*

I am a midwife but I have chosen not to share my midwifery skills in New Zealand because I am hurt beyond belief that I have had to fight for two years to return.

If you have read this email, for that I am thankful. I would appreciate to hear your response.

Nga mihi

The iron curtain around NZ borders finally lifted early March 2022. We could return and the isolation restrictions had finally been adapted to meet the coronavirus reality. Jeff and I passed the ultimate Coronavirus test by having a negative screen. I arrived in Aotearoa stunned, bruised from rejection and unsure of if I would fit. During my time as the midwife, I wondered if I had lost my joy for the profession. I had let go of so much that had been my life and I had embarked on a new chapter by organic means. Our first three months was spent letting the ghosts of our homelands settle. We introduced each other to our cousins and aunties. We met up with mutual friends from back in the day and introduced each other to others. We toured the length and breadth of the country and walked the mighty Milford Track. We both witnessed Jeff's daughter graduate to become a Barrister and Solicitor. He triumphed as a proud father. He had been an amazingly supportive father to his only daughter all her life, under exceptional challenges.

I am embarking on a new chapter in my life embracing the extreme cold and settling into the wee cottage in the Central Otago goldfields where my parents lived in the 1950's and retired back to in the 80s. I look out onto the cycle path and listen to the Teviot stream bubbling past on its final flow into Te mata au, the mighty Clutha river. There is no stress here. No demands. I don't have to be responsible for women and their babies.

Is it time to slow down? Time to settle, even?

I check my inbox and my travel agent has just contacted me, asking if I want to book my ticket back to London?

Hmm...

———

46   POST SCRIPT

My return to London eventually happened. It was like those dreams that linger between wakefulness and sleep, where my mind wandered through the possible thoughts and feelings that London would present when I got there. The excited anticipation of the flight was absent, whether real or imagined. I wondered if this had happened to all the travellers who had almost given up hope of returning to where their lives were before the world changed. Had everyone lost the joy of the adventures ahead? It was difficult to gauge the mood as I checked my luggage in at Dunedin Airport. Were people feeling downbeat?

I would be flying over 19,000km, spending 27.5 hours in the air and 10 hours of stopovers before landing. When I arrived at Heathrow airport, it felt familiar. However, it wasn't until the full plane load of passengers filed through passport control that the first hint that things had changed hit me. Staff shortages seemed to be the most common post-Covid issue. After standing and waiting for our luggage for three hours, no one got upset or had dramatic outbursts demanding information. We were all just resigned to the situation, although for me, I was so relieved to be here. My usual philosophical self-accepted the high possibility that my luggage, having been last seen in a domestic airport the furthest distance possible from Heathrow, too many days and hours ago, may not appear. But it did.

Covid is still around, and people are still isolating. However, Londoners' resilience doesn't seem to have been dampened. My time in London was like a see-saw of emotions. Anticipation as I returned to old haunts was met with wistful sadness, loss but resignation. Uncertainty of reactions when I visited old friends turned to comfortable catch-ups. The uncertainty of how the world had changed, saying goodbye to my former life and my former self, which I had held onto with an increasingly failing grasp while accidentally in Australia, was replaced with a settled soul.

Jet lag and sensory overload exhausted me, but I couldn't resist the feeling that I was home. That inescapable, intangible concept of home. Had there been a pandemic, lockdowns, deaths, PPE, border closures? When I looked around, it would appear not. Perhaps less crowding on the underground and signs to wear masks which were ignored by most gave the only clue. A few abandoned café signs were hanging in the streets, many replaced by bright energetic healthier take-out versions a few doors along. Bus routes had been rationalised and run less frequently, and alternative routes were in place.

The energy in London's Stansted airport was sober, but it was packed, and the food outlets were open for restricted hours and seemed to be taking turns at sharing the retail pound. Rome was still there, and so were the tourists. Mask-wearing was more noticeable but remained infrequent.

The Queen died at 15:10 BST on 8 September 2022 and was publicly announced at 18.30. I was at the NZ society summer drinks event in a boat club on the river Thames, surrounded by Antipodeans, when we absorbed the news. My Ngāti Rānana colleague and I sang the national anthem in Te Reo Māori and English. This was my London life. If I hadn't written this book, I could be excused for wondering if the Covid pandemic had actually happened.

NOTES

3. Storm

1. bikini options for men

4. Holiday in Australia

1. https://www.nma.gov.au/defining-moments/resources/national-apology

5. Small hospital bureaucracy

1. Australian for 'being unwell

8. Norseman or Horseman

1. Bogan- an uncouth or unsophisticated person regarded as being of low social status

10. Australia's longest straightest road

1. Australian for temporary, usually transportable dwelling.

13. Priscilla Queen of the Desert

1. https://en.wikipedia.org/wiki/Death_of_Azaria_Chamberlain

14. Quarantine In Alice Springs

1. Local aboriginal term for having a chat

22. Karlu Karlu - Getting away from it all

1. Australians tend to shorten words. Mozzies is short for mosquitoes
2. liquor

25. Tennant Creek Communities

1. The mourning period when a family member dies and all responsibilities that follow in accordance with traditional lore and custom
2. Northern Territory
3. Ethanol alcohol addiction
4. Aboriginal people use the word 'yarn' meaning 'chatted'

26. WA Border Opening

1. An extended family or community of related families who live together in the same area.
2. Triodia is a large genus of tussock forming grasses that are endemic to Australia, which is more commonly known as 'spinifex' and is often what people mean when they talk about spinifex and spinifex grass.

38. Wangkatjungka clients

1. The **redback spider** (*Latrodectus hasselti*), also known as the **Australian black widow**,[2][3][4] is a species of highly venomous spider believed to originate in South Australia or adjacent Western Australian deserts, but now found throughout Australia, Southeast Asia and New Zealand, with colonies elsewhere outside Australia.
   https://en.wikipedia.org/wiki/Redback_spider
2. King Edward Memorial Hospital in Perth. It is a specialised hospital primarily focused on maternity and women's health services.
   KEMH provides a range of services including prenatal care, childbirth, postnatal care, gynecological services, fertility treatment, and neonatal care.

39. ANZAC Day 2021

1. https://www.bl.uk/events/ngati-ranana-celebrating-60-years-of-maori-culture-in-london

40. Calling it a day

1. https://en.wikipedia.org/wiki/Stolen_Generations
2. The **Horizontal Falls**, or **Horizontal Waterfalls**, nicknamed the "**Horries**" and known as **Garaanngaddim** by the local Indigenous people, are an unusual natural phenomenon on the coast of the Kimberley region in Western Australia, where tidal flows cause waterfalls on the ebb and flow of each tide. The **Lalang-garram / Horizontal Falls Marine Park** is a protected area covering the falls and wider area.

https://en.wikipedia.org/wiki/Horizontal_Falls
3. A piece of turf cut out of the ground by a golf club in making a stroke or by a sports player's boot.

www.ingramcontent.com/pod-product-compliance
Lightning Source LLC
Chambersburg PA
CBHW011614290426
44110CB00021BA/2590